pretty
SANE

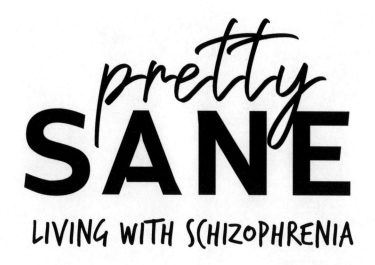

pretty SANE

LIVING WITH SCHIZOPHRENIA

NICOLA WALL

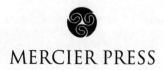

MERCIER PRESS

MERCIER PRESS

Cork

www.mercierpress.ie

ISBN: 978 1 78117 702 0

A CIP record for this title is available from the British Library.

Printed and bound in the EU.

FOR MICHAEL 'MOP' COLEMAN

Prologue

I always knew I was somewhat different without knowing exactly how. My earliest memory is being given a doll on my third birthday. One day around that time I am looking at a picture of a deer when it turns and runs towards me. There is a cushion with a peacock on it, it comes straight out at me. A woman in a painting turns her head to look at me, her eyes staring into mine until I squeak and run out of the room. It does not matter where I am – at home, my grandparents' house or my aunt's – pictures and paintings move around and then right themselves as soon as I attempt to show anyone. Whenever a picture turns itself into a television, I drag an adult by the hand to show them the magic painting, only to look like a liar when it fails to perform. I finally catch one in the act; my grandad John and I stand in front of the deer painting while it shakes its head and slowly stalks forward. 'The deer isn't moving, Nicola; it's just your imagination,' he tells me.

I often hear adults talking about my active imagination. No one ever believes that the things I see are real, even when

I show them. It takes me longer than it probably should to put two and two together and understand my experiences are somewhat unique. Like seeing the people who stand over my bed at night, or the woman outside my window who screams like a banshee. I spend most nights sleepless, staring at my curtains, waiting for them to open and reveal whoever is coming to visit me. I develop a fear of open curtains; you can never know who is standing at your window in the dead of night, waiting to come in.

Once I establish that some of my experiences are exclusive to me, I am more careful about keeping them to myself. Like the crows. I have a special bond with crows – they can communicate with me and I can talk back. They flock to me while I play in the garden and I tell them where to fly to next. In folklore, crows are seen as an omen for bad luck, disease or death. They are generally disliked, but I feel they are misunderstood. There is a lot more to them than people realise; for instance, they mate for life, they recognise human faces and they can change dialect. How lucky I am to be the human chosen to become queen of the crows. And who better to lead these intelligent, complex creatures than a curly haired little girl from Athlone with a lisp. Later in life, I learn that I am not the ruler of crows. I am a schizophrenic child experiencing her first psychotic delusion.

Next come the voices.

I cannot recall what my mind sounded like before. I don't remember silence, so I can't place when exactly the voices started. My head has always been full of noise like normal sounds that everyone experiences: street noise, cars, music, running water, general chatter. The only difference is that these sounds stay in my head, even when I am alone. I often compare it to being in a crowded restaurant: you can hear all the noise around you but you cannot specifically hear what people are saying unless you turn to the table beside you and listen to their conversation, or if someone from across the room shouts something particularly loud. That is the simplest way I can explain it; my mind sounds like a busy restaurant – and that's on a good day.

On a bad day, it's more like a crowded pub on a Saturday night. My voices can come from anywhere: a family member, friend, acquaintance, the person who serves me in the shop or the waiter who takes my food order; a lot of the time they come from the TV. They have different accents, emotions and personalities. If it comes from a person I know in real life, the voice is no reflection on them and has a completely different personality.

Going back to the beginning, as a child I never thought of all this noise as a bad thing. I didn't know what it sounded like in anyone else's head, so I assumed this was normal. Some voices come and go quicker than others; I might have a voice for a day or a year. There is only one voice that has consistently been in my head since the beginning and it belongs to Freddie. You are going to hear from Freddie a lot in this book.

Mental illness does not always fit the narrative that television, films and the media give it. All this nonsense of rocking back and forth in a padded cell, sitting on a park bench with your hood up, staring sadly into space or with your head in your hands – mental illness does not look like that. It often looks like a laughing, joyous person, the life and soul of the party. But what you don't see is the misery they feel inside. When you have a mental illness, you are expected to act like you don't have one for the most part.

The very first time I heard that we even have something called mental health was in fourth year of school, when a psychiatric nurse came to give us a talk. She told us about all the different signs and symptoms of anxiety and depression. Someone asked what it was like to work at a psychiatric hospital and I think her desire to come across as cool to a bunch of teenagers and impress us took over, because she spent the next twenty minutes telling us all funny stories about patients with bipolar disorder or schizophrenia and the crazy things they say and do. I sat there and thought, 'There is no way anyone can ever find out I'm like those people.' This was the first time I experienced the unwritten rule of mental health representation – depression and anxiety deserve sympathy, but the more severe illnesses are what the real crazy people have.

Thankfully not everyone feels like this. The truth is, no matter what your diagnosis, whether it's depression or borderline personality disorder, obsessive compulsive disorder, an eating disorder, post-traumatic stress or postnatal depression, bipolar disorder or anxiety, we are all in this together. We are the one in four, the ones who know how it feels to be trapped in our own minds, who struggle to make sense of our thoughts, who desperately want others to understand our invisible illness, who are so used to putting on a mask that we don't know how to take it off and be ourselves, who have a condition that affects every aspect of our lives, yet we are treated as though we could just get over it if we wanted to. I wrote this book for us.

I am not sure why you have chosen to read about my mental health experience. If you are looking for a self-help book, this isn't one. It's more like the opposite of one. I will tell you all the stupid, disastrous and dangerous ways I have coped with having a mental health problem and hopefully it will show you what not to do.

I want to show you, the reader, what it looks like inside my mind. I promise it won't all be doom and gloom. I may use words that could be deemed offensive – mental, crazy, schizo. These are all names that I have been called myself and I am a firm believer in taking ownership of the names people use against you, because if you embrace these yourself, they cannot be used to hurt you.

People might think that since I have schizoaffective disorder it means I'm mental, and they are kind of right. Maybe I am mental, but I have been mental for a very long time, and somewhere along the way, I got good at it. I have learned how to build a great life, how to be happy and how to live with a lifelong, incurable mental illness. This may not be a self-help book, but I will try to share a few lessons I have learned. By the way, I have changed the names of some people in this story because we wouldn't want to upset anyone, now, would we? This is my truth of how my life with schizoaffective disorder has been so far. This is my experience of mental illness and my journey of learning how to be mental.

Chapter 1

From the beginning, Freddie manages to be both a help and a hindrance. He is loud, brash and often obnoxious. He is strongly opinionated and judgemental, but he has a sweet side too. He is with me through good times and bad. His American twang bounces around my head, commenting on all that goes on around me. I live with my parents and my older brother, Jamie; he likes them all for the most part, which makes life easier for me. My dad's parents live next door, and they are a big part of my life, along with my aunt Sylvia and grandaunt Shelia. Despite my secret superpowers and the scary things I see, I am fairly content.

My world is turned upside down, however, when the bad woman comes along. I hate her. I can take banshees screaming and the people who climb in my window, but she is the worst. The most horrible thing of all is she doesn't seem to be like the others. My family appear to be able to see her and talk to her too. She is nice as pie when in the presence of others but cruel and nasty behind closed doors. She likes me, though. She even wants us to be friends; she tells me that she can be my mummy.

But I already have one of those and I love her very much, so that won't be happening.

Freddie hates the bad woman too. He warns me whenever she is near: *Stay away from the bad woman. She wants to steal you. She wants to take everything*.

The bad woman disappears one day. I ask about her, but no one will tell me where she went. She is just another part of my imagination. Like the faceless man, who hurts me and touches me in places he shouldn't. I need to stop making people up; my imagination is dangerous and it upsets everyone.

Everyone is sad all of a sudden, especially my mam. She tells me we are going to move away from Athlone, though we can still visit. We will be living in a new house by the sea, in a town called Dungarvan in Co. Waterford.

I am overcome with happiness; the faceless man and the bad woman will never find me there.

Freddie: *I thought they weren't real?*

'I know they're not, but they still feel real,' I tell him in my head.

I don't need to speak out loud to communicate with Freddie, or any of the other voices, although most of them don't listen to me anyway.

Freddie: *Alright then, you weirdo. How are we feeling about starting a new school?*

I am due to start first class when we make the move to our new home. I tell Freddie how excited I am about it.

Freddie: *Really? Sounds terrifying to me. You should be scared; what if everyone hates you?*

Sometimes Freddie can be a bit on the negative side.

I become more aware every day of how far behind I am. I watch my peers race ahead of me while I struggle to keep up and fit in with them. Jamie is smart and talented. He's good at music and computers. I don't feel like I'm good at anything. It seems like everyone has something, but I can't even keep up with the simple things.

The only skill I seem to have is that I can write with both hands. I switch from left to right and back again, whatever hand gets to the pencil first. I colour better with the left, while I struggle to keep in between the lines with my right, though I do have a firmer grip with my right hand. I see nothing wrong with this. Ambidextrous, Mam calls it, which sounds cool. I don't foresee the issue of elbows. Teacher puts lefties on the left so they don't elbow the righties while they work. Teacher is not impressed. She tells me to stick to the right – calmly, at first – but with each new day I keep forgetting. I do it naturally without thinking.

There is another problem. When I pick up a pencil and try to form the words, they come out all squiggly. Mam gets me pencil grips, but they don't help. Teacher gets more upset by the day. We establish what the problem is: I cannot hold the pencil properly. I am shown how but it doesn't make any sense to me. I can't write that way either and I forget how my fingers are supposed to wrap around it. Teacher hits me over the knuckles with a ruler repeatedly.

'Go on, Nicola. Write. I've shown you a million times; it's not hard,' she screams and growls and spits.

'Stupid girl,' I hear her mutter under her breath.

Freddie: *She's the stupid one. How does she expect you to write with your hand shaking? A hand will do that, you know, after you beat it with a ruler. Idiot.*

It is no good; I can't do it. I am quickly learning that I can't do anything. I leave my homework in school and my schoolwork at home. I forget my lunch. I don't understand how numbers work. I cannot memorise. I can't run fast or catch a ball. I walk into things. I drop everything. Stupid, useless and thick are words I hear a lot. Along with 'What's wrong with Nicola?'

The assessments start. I sit in many different offices where they ask the same questions and make me do tests.

It always goes the same way. They speak to me like I'm a baby or as if I am too slow to understand them.

I recall one particular appointment clearly. I sit on my hands to stop them from shaking and ticking. Apparently flapping your hands is not a normal thing to do, and I have been trying to be good. Adults get upset or annoyed when I flap or rock back and forth. I am expected to sit still. This is what people do, no one else seems to share my urge to shake, move, kick and pace. All the other children in my class can sit perfectly still without trying. For me, staying stationary is like a form of torture. It pleases people, though, so I pretend I am playing a game of statues for as long as I can until my body caves in and starts moving uncontrollably.

Freddie: *I think this is the part where she says what's wrong with you. At least we'll know then. They might leave you alone.*

The woman is explaining to my mother that I have slow cognitive functioning. I have poor concentration and memory. No surprises there. Everyone says I am away with the fairies and in my own little world.

This isn't true. They all think I can't pay attention, but they don't understand the rules. If someone is telling me something I tune out and listen to the voices, but I'm still paying attention, just in a different way. She is right in one sense, though: I may not be able to recall the pictures or numbers she showed me on the worksheet last week as part of her tests. I was concentrating on other things. I may not remember the boring illustrations and figures, but I can remember that she was wearing brown trousers, a white shirt and a yellow jacket. Her hair was pushed behind her right ear but hanging loose over her left. She had a blue pen, whereas this week it's black. I know exactly where each object was positioned on her desk compared to how they are arranged today. I know the name and author of every book on the shelves in her office. I can see the ones she reads regularly versus the ones that have sat there for a long time gathering dust. I see the *Handbook of Psychological and Educational Assessment of Children* has been moved from the second to the third shelf since our last appointment.

I am frustrated when they say I can't remember things.

Freddie: *Will you come back; you're missing everything here.*

The lady is still droning on about my shortcomings 'tricky one to diagnose' … 'still very young' … 'I know it's difficult'. My mother is hanging on her every word, of course, always wanting to know how to fix me.

The lady says something interesting then. She explains how the tests show a pattern; I find easy tasks to be difficult, while difficult tasks come easily to me.

Freddie: *Now there is a thought. I think that makes sense, don't you? She's very nice but I don't like her teeth, they are way too big for her mouth. Tell her to fix them.*

Some of the other voices chime in on the teeth discussion. I am still thinking about the easy/difficult thing. This is true. I know what she means; I can understand stuff but it's all backwards. Everyone in my class can tell the time now. They just look at the clock with the hands and they have it. I don't know how they do this; I can only tell what time it is by looking at a digital twenty-four-hour clock.

Silly little things like this are always being commented on. This woman has worked it out. What a clever doctor.

Freddie: *Her teeth are still rotten, though.*

The conversation has moved on to the fidgeting and rocking. She has no explanation for my excessive movements. They have a name, though: motor tics. I might grow out of them, she says.

I see so many people like this lady that they start to blur into one. I see a speech therapist, who tries to teach me how to talk properly. A psychologist to work out why I'm so sad. A doctor to figure out why I don't sleep. Everyone wants to know what's wrong with Nicola. If I wasn't before, I am now well aware that I am not normal. And being normal seems to be the most important thing in the world.

I want to be left alone. I don't like when people touch me, hugs make my skin crawl. I don't like people in general, there are far too many of them and they are far too loud. I want to understand things but I can only focus on what interests me. I become obsessed with things easily, whether it's a movie, a band, a book, a thought or a feeling. I don't like how some textures feel, like cotton and ribbons. I don't like food; only certain types and it has to look exactly the way I want it to before I'll even consider eating it. I get frustrated and confused when things are not how they are supposed to be. I scream and cry and kick. Yet I wish more than anything to be normal. I want to be like the other girls. I don't know what's wrong with me. Maybe it isn't me, after all, maybe the voices in my head are broken and everybody else's voices work properly so they're normal and not a freak like me.

Freddie: *Don't blame me, I'm the brains behind this operation. It's not my fault you can't make friends.*

'That's not true. I have friends,' I tell him.

Freddie: *You sure about that, sunshine?*

He has a point. I don't fit in all that well. I am shy and quiet, and walking around the playground in circles, shaking a pencil to calm myself down, doesn't exactly attract my class-mates to me. I can't help it, though. I need a physical outlet, otherwise the motor tics just get worse. But I do have friends, despite what Freddie says; we are at that age where weird isn't the worst thing you can be.

There is another issue: recognising faces. I know what people look like, I know what my parents look like and my brother. Almost all of my family have faces that I can remember easily, most of the time. But when my head is in the bad place and

I cannot think clearly, their faces get muddled up. I can make out people's eyes and ears and noses and mouths, but then I forget them; they all look the same to me most of the time, even people at school whom I see nearly every day. I try to remember them, but when I see them again the following morning, they look entirely different to the picture I had in my head.

The faceless man was not the same as this, though; he had no face at all. He looked like a shadow, a shadow that came to see me and made me scared of everything after he had gone. I never looked at him properly, except for one time when I was feeling brave. He wasn't as mean as I thought he would be. He was actually nice to me, apart from when he would hurt me. He gave me cake once. I knew he was a bad man, but once I listened to him and did whatever he wanted it wasn't so bad. He told me if I turned and faced the wall it would be over quickly; he preferred when I didn't look at his eyes. That was easy because I couldn't make them out anyway.

I hope he is gone for good now; even if he is only someone who lived inside my brain, he still felt like a person to me and I don't want him to ever seem real again.

HOW TO BE MENTAL TIP 1

I always get in trouble for forgetting things like my lunch or my schoolbag but there is another time of forgetting. Sometimes you need to forget on purpose, take the thoughts and push them far away. You can think about them every now and then, but not all the time. Some things are best forgotten.

Chapter 2

My grandaunt Shelia is one of the few people who never seems to have an issue with me getting lost in my imagination. Whenever I stay with her, she takes out my favourite toy of all time. A wooden plank, which I call 'the board'. It's not just any old plank of wood: it can be a table, a bus, a train, a house or a chalkboard. Shelia watches the news a lot. I write down the stories and set up my news desk with the board and read out all manner of current affairs to her little Yorkshire terrier.

My grandad doesn't think there is anything wrong with how I am either. John doesn't like people. He hates socialising and small talk. We get along quite well because of this.

My family is small compared to others; I only have a handful of cousins. I always wanted to be part of a larger family. When my parents tell me they are having a baby, I am so excited to become a big sister. I just cannot wait to not be the youngest any more. Jamie is alright, but he likes to torment me whenever the mood takes him. He was so disappointed at me being a girl and not the little brother he had dreamed of that he called me Christopher for the first years of my life. He also learned the Dracula theme song on the keyboard and came up with an elaborate stunt involving fake blood that had me convinced for longer than I care to admit that he was an actual vampire. He reads my diary and generally harasses me, but we do band together when needs be. Like when Mam bans us from watching some of our favourite TV shows after school because she read somewhere that shows like *California Dreams* and *Saved by the Bell* will corrupt us somehow. We stage a protest in a show of solidarity, along with a presentation of how *Boy Meets World* is important to our emotional development. It's nice having a big brother, but I am looking forward to moving up the ranks.

Freddie is not so impressed. He hates babies. I hear a baby's cry in my head sometimes, which always sets him off.

Freddie: *Make it stop. Nicola. Tell the baby to shut up. I don't like this; you know I don't like when it does this. Nicola. Nicola, are you listening to me?*

'I have to listen to it too, you have more control than I do, you tell the baby to stop.'

Freddie: *Don't be ridiculous. If I could shut it up I would.*

Freddie has always been the main communicator with the voices. I cannot talk to most of them directly, but I can pass messages through him occasionally. This makes him feel important and does his already over-inflated ego no favours. I have little to no control over Freddie or the other voices; I am not sure whether this is because of my usual incompetence or just the way it is for everyone.

I wonder where my parents are when our neighbour wakes me up.

Freddie: *Probably gone to have the sprog.*

'You're getting a little brother or sister today,' the neighbour says.

I can hardly contain my excitement in school and tell everyone my news. Someone asks me will I be jealous and if I'm sad that I won't be the youngest any more. But I only feel utter joy when I imagine being a big sister. I will be eight years older than the baby, so I can help look after it and when I'm a teenager I can babysit. I think of chubby little cheeks and tiny hands. I picture my sibling toddling around, smiling, laughing and all the cuddles. I plan trips with it in my head, going to the playground and the cinema. I wonder will Mam let me push the buggy. I don't care if the baby is a boy or a girl, I just want to protect it and look out for it.

Stephen is born on 15 September. I am elated. My dad comes home, sits with me on the stairs and tells me that my brother is sick and needs an operation to get better. He cannot have the operation until he is in a stable condition, so we have to wait. It takes me a while to ask the question. I'm sitting at the kitchen table with my neighbour's sons, drawing pictures. I'm drawing one of Stephen to bring to the hospital. My dad stands over my shoulder, watching me draw the little baby.

'What will happen if he can't have the operation?'

He leans down and whispers, 'Well then, he'll die.'

Oh, that is not what I was expecting. I didn't think babies could die.

Freddie: *You should add some wings to him for when he goes to live in the clouds.*

My parents want life to go on as normally as possible for Jamie and me. We head into school the next day. I'm scared. My dad is acting as if everything is fine. I miss my mam and wonder if she is alright. Is she sad? Or scared? My teacher asks me if my little sibling has been born. I tell her he was but he is sick. Later, I cry in the toilets. She finds me and I tell her I'm afraid he's going to die.

'Of course he's not going to die, don't be silly,' she says.

She says a lot of things. About how babies are born sick all the time and I shouldn't worry about something that hasn't happened yet.

I don't think she meant to say the word yet. I think she wants me to be okay and go back to class. I know I'm supposed to be comforted by her words, tell her she's right and put a smile on my face. I'm not good at knowing what is the right thing to do or say. I get an awful lot wrong, especially when it comes to talking to people, but one thing I have noticed is how people always want you to be happy. Which sounds nice, but it's not so nice when you find it hard to be happy. In this case, the teacher gets frustrated with me. She stops using her soft voice and gets cross with me. That's what they do, they get angry when you're sad. It's easier to pretend sometimes. So, with great effort, I do.

I keep on pretending when we go to see him. I want to get him something at the gift shop. I look at all the teddies. I pick up a black bunny rabbit.

Freddie: *No, not that one.*

I put it back and put my hand on a light-brown one.

Freddie: *That's the one. What you gonna call him?*

'Bunnyfluff.' He has a fluffy tail.

Freddie: *Not very imaginative but okay.*

When we walk into the room all I can see are machines, some of which are bigger than me, and cots with lots of wires. It takes me a moment to realise the wires are attached to something. Or someone. There are tiny babies in each cot. We wash our hands before putting on plastic aprons. We have to do this to protect the tiny sick babies from outside germs.

Dad brings me over to one of the tiny sick babies. There are bubbles of saliva coming out of his mouth, in a gap between the baby's lips and the tube going into his mouth. His chest is moving up and down really fast. He is pink.

That's him then. My little brother.

Freddie: *Is it supposed to look like a wrinkly old man?*

I show Mam Bunnyfluff. She asks me if I want to put him in beside Stephen. I stare at the tiny sick baby.

Freddie: *What if you didn't wash your hands properly and there's germs still on them? Imagine what that could do to him.*

'Go on, it's alright,' Mam says.

My dad lifts me up so I can reach properly. I touch his cheek first, then his hand. It's so light that, at first, I think I am imagining it.

'He's squeezing my finger.'

'He must know you're his big sister,' Mam says.

I look at him in wonder. I always wanted to be a big sister, but not like this. He is perfect.

An alarm goes off on his machine.

Freddie: *Jesus Christ, you've killed him.*

'It's alright. That happens all the time,' the nurse says, seeing my panicked face as she fiddles with one of the machines.

Freddie: *She's only saying that to make you feel better.*

Stephen is going to be okay. That's what my dad says anyway. I hear him say it all the time. He is going to have the operation and come home.

'When Stephen is in his buggy can I push it?' I ask him.

'Of course you can.'

'And can I give him his bottle?'

'Of course you can.'

'When I'm older, can I babysit? Like, properly.'

'Yes, when you're older.'

I ask him questions like this on the many car journeys between home in Dungarvan, Athlone and Crumlin Hospital in Dublin. I go to school most of the time. It's usually on the weekends that we stay in Athlone, going back and forth to the hospital. Stephen sleeps most of the time when we visit. All the machines whirl around him but he just lies there, blowing his bubbles. Bunnyfluff sits beside him.

'He'll keep you safe,' I whisper to Stephen as I say goodbye one day.

I go to school and tell everyone how my brother is getting better. I write stories and draw pictures; I staple them all together to make books for him to read when he's older. He might love to read like me. I have a lot of books but they might be for girls more than boys so he can read my original stories instead.

It is time to go see him again. We arrive late in the evening to John and Phyllis' house in Athlone; she's made up a bed for me. It's in the scary room. The one where I used to see the monsters the most. My mam knows how I feel about it; she usually makes sure I get a different room, but she is staying in the hospital with Stephen. I don't want to make a fuss. I could never explain to Phyllis why I don't like that room. My mam gets it only because she understands things that most people don't. I have to be brave, I'm a big sister now, after all. I can't teach Stephen not to be afraid of things if I am.

I lie in bed and stare at the curtains. I wait for them to come visit me. They always come out from behind the curtains. I listen for them. I wish they would hurry up and appear. I want to get it over with. They haven't visited me in a long time. Sometimes, I think they might actually be nice. Maybe they just want to be my friend. I wonder if they ever visit Jamie. Or if John and Phyllis have ever seen them – most likely, since they live in the house. I don't believe adults when they blame my imagination. They must be one of those things that you're supposed not to talk about, like what your voices say.

Morning comes and no dark figures visited me. The room is bright. I slept here for the first time in years and nothing bad happened. I get up and make my way down the hall. My mother comes out of the sitting room. I haven't seen her outside of the hospital since Stephen was born.

This can only mean one thing. They are home. Stephen is better.

'Nic, I'm so sorry, but Stephen went up to heaven last night.'

HOW TO BE MENTAL TIP 2

You can't be positive all the time. You need to think of the worst scenario too, otherwise it hurts even more when your heart breaks because you didn't see it coming.

Mam says it is important that we see him, she wants everyone to see him. He was a person. He lived, if only for a short while. Everyone should see him and say goodbye, like at most funerals.

He is in a little white coffin wrapped up in his blanket. His eyes are open. The mass takes place in the hospital chapel. Lots of our friends and family are there. When it's over they leave the room and it's just the five of us left. I wrote him a letter, and so I put it inside the coffin. I'm too selfish to put Bunnyfluff in with him. I want to keep the teddy for myself. Stephen lived and died with the cuddly toy beside him. If I keep it, I'll always have a part of him. He won't need it, anyway. This is just his body. His soul will go somewhere else. My mam explained that to me. Even though I understand this, I still panic when they close the coffin.

We drive to the cemetery in Athlone. Our parents sit in the front of the car. The white coffin sits in the middle between Jamie and I in the back seat. The four of us carry the coffin to the grave. I won't see him again. This is the last time and I am not ready. I want to scream as they lower it. He won't like it down there. The hardest part is seeing my mam so sad all the time. She talks about her dad a lot – he died when she was young.

A lady approaches her in town one day, 'Oh did you have the baby?'

'Yes. He died.'

I like how she says it. I don't like when people don't say what they mean. People keep saying we lost Stephen, like he was a set of keys or something. Or that he passed away. But he died. I don't see why we have to use ridiculous phrases to make dying sound nicer. Death isn't nice.

Freddie: *I don't know why you're all making such a huge deal anyway. It's not like you ever knew him. You can't miss someone you never really knew.*

'I hate you, Freddie.'

Chapter 3

When I get to the age of ten I really start to hate myself. I dislike being different and don't understand what it is that makes me unusual in the first place. I hate myself for being stupid, ugly, fat and, most of all, useless. I can't be normal, I have tried and tried; even if I could just pretend to be like everyone else it could help. Faking being normal doesn't work when I can't stay still. It's like I have all this extra energy stored up in my bones and if I don't let it out, I twitch or tic. The only way to use it all up is to give in to the impulses, so I pace up and down, shake my hands or an object and get some relief.

'Hey.'

'Freddie?'

'Not Freddie.'

'Oh.'

'See that knife? Pick it up.'

'Which one?' I pull one from the knife block on the counter in the kitchen. 'This?'

'No, stupid, that's a carving knife.'

I pace around the kitchen. I don't want to make the voice mad. I pick up another one.

'*Use it.*'

There is a moment, a split second where I ask myself the obvious question: why? But I ignore my thoughts, I don't need to use my own mind sometimes. I put it to my arm and cut. It only hurts a little. I can handle it.

Freddie: *Excuse me, what do you think you're doing?*

'Cutting my arm.'

Freddie: *Oh right. Carry on then.*

Blood starts to seep out. I am not pressing down hard. I don't want to hurt myself properly, but now that I have started, I want to see what happens.

Freddie: *Yeah, you know what, kid, I don't think you should do that any more.*

'Okay.'

I go to wash the knife.

Freddie: *You've got to stop listening to what other people in your head say, okay, kid? It can be dangerous. Only listen to me; you like me, yeah? I'm your favourite.*

'No, I don't like you.'

Freddie: *But –*

'But I'll listen to you anyway.'

HOW TO BE MENTAL TIP 3

If you hear bad things in your head, it's a good idea to stop and question them before you believe everything they say.

I am trying to be more responsible, especially now that I am a big sister. My little brother Gary was born a year after Stephen died. He is only starting toddlerhood now, but he is already wild. Having a younger sibling is everything I thought it would be so far; I get to do all the things we missed out on with Stephen and everyone is less sad since Gary came along. My parents keep reminding me that I have to set a good example for him. I'm not too worried about that yet. Gary doesn't care if I forget my homework or that I'm not very good at socialising. He only cares that I push him on the swings and know all the words to 'Bob the Builder'.

Speaking of homework, times have changed nowadays I think (hope) in the school system. There seems to be more understanding in the idea that school is not for everyone and that not all children learn the same way. School was certainly never right for me, though, particularly in 1990s Ireland, where learning difficulties were barely acknowledged.

Most teachers seem to dismiss me, but there are some exceptions. For two years, I have a teacher who behaves differently from most of the adults in my life so far. She doesn't make me feel stupid.

I wanted to be a journalist or a writer until I was told I would be too shy for journalism. I took this to heart and stopped writing my silly stories, interviewing my family members for my daily news reports. But this teacher spots it, through all my failings at maths and Irish and history and every other subject. She notices that I like to write, and encourages me to be creative about it again. She shows my parents my writing and they're proud. She teaches a speech and drama class outside of school, which I join. I love the drama part; pretending to be other people gives me an escape from being me. I learn public speaking, which I'm not actually bad at. I enjoy it so much that I sign up for other drama clubs. I even get the lead role in some productions. There is something about standing up on a stage in front of an audience that clears my mind: I focus on remembering my lines and the noise in my head fades into the background. It is not some big turning point or breakthrough for me, it doesn't make me normal or all the things I wish I could be, but, for a few years, it makes me a tiny bit happier.

The big moment of realisation happens in the playground, when I am twelve. I am talking to Freddie, worrying about how badly I am doing in school, about not fitting in and why I can't be like everyone else. I watch other kids make friends easily. They can hold conversations for long periods of time, they don't get distracted mid-sentence and trail off, they don't pace up and down or have to go to a corner and be by themselves when everything around them gets too much, when it gets too loud.

And there it is.

Loud. It doesn't get too loud.

Freddie: *Yeah? Keep going, you're getting somewhere.*

'They aren't like me. Everyone else, they can't hear what I can hear. It's you, it's you, Freddie, you are what makes me different. All of them, they don't have a Freddie. They don't hear any loud noises, they don't hear.'

Freddie: *Hear what? You're nearly there.*

'Voices. They don't hear voices.'

Freddie: *You got it. Gold star.*

The change in my awareness makes me feel more of a freak than ever. I cannot understand how this works. If they don't hear voices, what do they hear? Do their minds just sound empty? Who tells them what to do? How do they make decisions? The biggest question of all: are they just by themselves all the time? My family, my classmates, my teachers, the people on the street – when they are in a room with no other people in it, that's just all there is, they are alone. This doesn't make sense.

Freddie: *Seems like it's the case, though. It's the only explanation that works.*

'How did you get into my head in the first place?'

Freddie: *I've always been here.*

'No, but how did you, I don't know, start, I suppose? Were you here when I was born?'

Freddie: *No. Well, I don't remember that far back. I was always just here from when we were in Athlone. I can only recall the same things that you can. I can't see into the future either before you start getting any mad ideas. I stay in the present, just like you.*

'What about when you go away? When I don't hear you, where are you then?'

Freddie: *I don't know, I'm just here I guess and then I'm not, I am nowhere and then I am with you. There's nothing else. I only exist in your mind; I suppose that's the only way I can explain it.*

'So, I made you up then?'

Freddie: *Well, yeah, kid, I guess you did.*

'Like I made them up. The faceless man, the bad woman. Are you like them?'

Freddie: *No. I don't know. You're confusing me now. Are we talking about how real I am or how real everything else is?*

'The other voices. Did I make them up too? That doesn't make any sense at all. I can't control what any of you say; if I made you, why don't you just say what I think?'

Freddie: *Now I'm really confused.*

That makes two of us. I am lost, truly lost in the world. Freddie cannot shed any light on my situation. I don't know what is real and what is not any more. Is this why I am so slow, or why I can't recognise people's faces properly?

One thing is clear, no one can know. This is far worse than I thought. Hearing voices is very bad, I know this, and if I say anything, I will only make everything worse. If I want to be normal, I have to keep my mouth shut about all of it. As far as the child psychologists know, there are no voices in my head. I have mentioned them before in passing, when I thought everyone could hear them, but I never used the word voices. No wonder they think I'm strange, but they probably didn't understand what I meant whenever I said there was too much noise in my mind. I think I have gotten away with it. They are more focused on my other problems: the tics, my short attention span, how overwhelmed I get by my surroundings, my lack of social skills, the obsessive behaviour.

I feel like the list of what's wrong with me is getting longer all the time. I do their tests and answer their questions. In the middle of it all, I end up in hospital after being out sick from school for weeks. They do tests in there too; I'm underweight and they think I have some kind of stomach problem. When I am discharged, they put it down to some mystery virus.

No one notices that I have been getting sick on purpose. I figured out how to do it a while ago. I don't like sticking my fingers down my throat much, so when I don't feel like that there is another way. I eat until I get sick or eat the foods that came up in the allergy test Mam brought me to. Either way it works. I get some of the rottenness out of my body and you can see my bones now. It is not as good as cutting, but I am still not very good at that. I need more practice. I'm learning that you can do pretty much anything without anyone noticing, if you are quiet enough about it.

In the end, ADHD is what I am diagnosed with – attention deficit hyperactivity disorder – and slowed cognitive functioning. My parents decide not to put me on medication. The doctor says we can explore other options, such as autism or dyspraxia, later on, but I am still young and he is sure that I don't want to be stuck with a label.

No one asks me if I want to know what is wrong with me. I don't get to choose to go on medication, even if it might make me normal. None of it makes sense to me really. If I have autism, I have autism. If I have dyspraxia or ADHD then I have them. Surely you don't get to pick and choose which conditions you have or don't have? If the boy in my school who has diabetes decides he doesn't want a label, does he just decide not to have diabetes any more? The day I'm diagnosed with ADHD is also the last time I see a child psychologist. I am a case that has been cracked, so now there is no need to see me any more.

Chapter 4

I am nervous but hopeful starting secondary school. It feels as though it could be a fresh start, though at the same time my track record for doing well at school or making friends is not great. Well, the making friends part is not too bad but maintaining the friendship is where I struggle. I crave alone time. When it is just me and Freddie, I feel safe; he can be insensitive, cruel and cold, but he understands me in a way no one else can. Other people pale in comparison. With others, I have to explain myself, get to know them, let them inside a bit so they can understand me better. With Freddie, I don't have to hide anything, there is no need to pretend, he doesn't expect me to be normal. And I have decided that, in secondary school, I am going to be normal, even if I'm not.

I am slowly coming to terms with my uniqueness. It still puzzles me how it works. How other people's minds sound without voices; I imagine that it must come with a level of isolation worse than anything I have ever experienced. As I am trying to comprehend this, I am also realising that there are more differences between myself and others. The biggest one being mind reading, a skill everyone around me seems to have that I don't possess. Like for the voices, I don't know how it works. I am becoming suspicious that everyone around me has known about the voices all along. Sending me to all of those doctors, changing the subject whenever I tried to talk about the bad woman, dismissing the faceless man as an imaginary character and all the conversations – the 'What's wrong with Nicola?' conversations, as Freddie and I call them – even those are just distractions. They have been misleading me all this time, keeping the focus on silly things like ADHD and learning disorders, while all along they could listen into my mind and hear my thoughts. If they can hear what I am thinking, they must be able to hear the voices too. No wonder they think I am a freak.

Freddie and I have been practising techniques to keep people out of our head. We try making loud noises or being really quiet. I keep my thoughts neutral about other people so as not to offend them. Freddie isn't very good at that, but we are a work in progress.

We meet lots of new people in my new school. It is exhausting, trying to make friends with people while figuring out their motive. Maybe not everyone can mind read? It could just be a half-the-population scenario; in that case I am getting angry at people for reading my mind without my permission when they aren't. There could be others, I think, just like I was, going about their day, unaware that they are surrounded by people who are listening to their thoughts. Perhaps I should warn them.

I befriend a group of girls; it feels nice to be part of something. I have had friends before, of course, but none of those friendships ended very well. Normal girls have a group of friends, this is good. I am lucky that they have chosen me. I don't fit too well in their circle, but they keep me around nonetheless. It's nice to feel normal, even if it isn't real. We go to each other's houses, hang around town aimlessly, go to the cinema, go shopping, talk about boys, borrow each other's clothes. All normal things. Then there's the alcohol, smoking and doing things with boys that we're probably far too young to do, but that's what everyone does. And one thing I have learned about normal people: they do what everyone else does. If you just go along with it and do what everyone is doing, well then, you'll blend right in.

When I get too comfortable being normal, the girls are quick to remind me that I'm not like them. They make fun of me a lot. I am weird, I say strange things, they don't like my accent and even the way I walk is wrong. The thing they hate most about me is how I tune out of conversations and come back to them confused. That really gets under their skin. I'm talking to Freddie in my head, but this is why I can't tell anyone about him, they would really hate me then. I am slowly learning that there is a lot of hatred in friendships; one day you are best friends and the next they don't want anything to do with you. I don't fancy boys, or even girls, but everyone else does, so I pretend. If I don't, the girls make fun of me. Normal girls have boyfriends, so I get one. I don't like him very much and he doesn't like me outside of what I can give him. We're just using each other, but it keeps the girls off my back.

I manage to hold on to my first group of friends for two whole years. It ends badly. By the end, they are barely even pretending to like me. After the boyfriend and I break up and he starts going out with one of the other girls, I take my leave.

It's the summertime, so all it takes is one phone call and I am enrolled in another school without having to make any kind of dramatic exit from my old one. I can just softly slip away, not appearing in September, and they can forget about me. They seem happy with that. I know those girls all grew up to be genuinely nice people. In an all-girls school, bitchiness is inevitable. I was no saint myself, but for the most part I think I was an easy target and if it was going to be anyone getting laughed at and mocked, it was going to be me. For someone as unusual as me, I think I actually escaped being bullied really badly.

HOW TO BE MENTAL TIP 4

Not everyone is going to like you. You won't like everyone either. Some people are just not for you, so trying to force them to understand you will never work. Neither of you is right or wrong. Don't waste each other's time or try to bring someone down because they see the world differently. Criticising a person's entire being is not going to change them into the person you want them to be, and you are not doing them any favours. It won't make them like you more, it just makes them like themselves less.

That summer, not for the first time, I find myself friendless and alone. I go to Athlone to stay with John, Phyllis and Shelia until it's time to start my new school. I come up with a plan. Freddie says he will help me. I have a whole summer ahead of me before I start my new school. I have tried to fake being normal before without much success, but this time I am determined. And I have a secret weapon: *Big Brother*. The reality TV show where bunches of people from all walks of life are thrown into a house, voting each other out one by one until there is a winner. It is essentially a popularity contest and at this point in time it's one of the biggest shows on television. I take in their conversations, their arguments; I watch how they form friendships, how they get along living in such an enclosed environment. I observe their reactions to what goes on around them; I take in their facial expressions and how they each show emotion, happiness, anger; I get a better understanding of social cues, body language, vocal tones and what they mean.

Now, I know learning social norms from a crowd of eccentric wannabe celebrities acting up to the camera may not seem like the best idea, but you have to work with what you have. *Big Brother* featured a twenty-four-hour live feed and I had tapes of the few previous series too. Funnily enough, it worked. The show taught me how to communicate better. I practised in the mirror, with Freddie shouting at me whenever I made a mistake. It didn't make me normal, but it showed me how to blend in and, at that point in my life, that was all I needed.

HOW TO BE MENTAL TIP 5
Fake it until you make it.

My new school ends up being far more successful. I make friends who are not like the ones from my old school; they actually seem to like me. We tell each other everything. Well, they tell me things; I am as selective as ever in what I share. Voices and mind reading are obvious no-go areas. Now, I will warn you, these friends at times are going to sound like not-so-good people. What is important to remember is that you are only hearing my side of the story. I'm sure if you could hear theirs I would probably look like the bad guy. They may have let me down spectacularly in the end, as you will find out, but the truth is, they never really knew me. No one did. I created a fake persona that got me through most of my teenage years. I pretended not to be psychotic, which I am sure most people in my situation would do. But I took it a step further than that.

That summer spent learning 'how to be normal' via *Big Brother* had done me a world of good. I fitted in with people much better, but what you need to know is I turned up at my new school as a completely different person. My previous friends had mocked my accent, so I'd practised saying different words over and over until I had a new, almost entirely different accent. I had changed the way I walked, smiled, how I reacted to things. I literally stored away my rehearsed facial expressions, ready to consciously use the appropriate one. I know now how odd that might seem. After all, I perfected my confused expression while watching Jade Goody find out that Rio de Janeiro was a city and not a person. I understand looking concerned when someone tells you their cat is sick and then looking happy when they tell you Fluffy is doing better might seem like basic human behaviour to most people, but, for me, it was something I needed to figure out by watching one of the first reality TV shows. I dread to think what would have happened had the Kardashians been around – I can only imagine what sort of character I would have created for myself then. Overall, it was a bit out there, but it worked. Yes, I was still a little off, but I passed myself off as a 'normie' for the most part.

***

The next few years are relatively uneventful. My ability to compartmentalise helps me to hide my ever-developing mental health problems. As I have said before, a lot of the time, my thinking doesn't make sense (but you might have noticed that already). I think everyone can read my mind, but at the same time I am giving myself a pat on the back for hiding the voices. I think being psychotic is a reasonable explanation for my lack of logic.

More theories begin to pop into my head. I start being more aware of security cameras. Then, when camera phones become a thing, I worry about them too. I figure there are listening devices planted in my room and nothing I say or do is ever private. Being followed is another fear of mine. If I walk around a shop and the security guard (who realistically is just bored off his trolley and hoping I'll try to lift something to liven up his day) has his eye on me, I think that's it, he is one of them. I am not sure who 'they' are, but both my mind and the voices refer to 'them', and 'they' are out to get me.

I tear through food, cutting it up into tiny little pieces. I am usually looking for signs that it has been poisoned, but sometimes I search for daddy long legs. A voice mentioned one day that there could be one stuck in my food and so I get a complex about it. Why someone would want to spike my food or put in a daddy long legs of all things is not what I ask myself; if a voice puts an idea into my head I believe it without question.

It gets madder than that. I start to think that inanimate objects are alive and I can talk to them. You know the first time you see *Toy Story* and then afterwards you sit in your room wondering if all your toys are in freeze mode but come alive when you're away? It's a bit like that except I am fifteen and should know that the kitchen utensils don't have feelings.

One of my most embarrassing memories is befriending a shampoo bottle. It is the brand Sunsilk and it must give me the strong, healthy hair it promised, because I grow rather fond of it. I talk to it, put it into bed at night and generally see it as a companion. I can't remember what became of that bottle – I probably moved on to the conditioner counterpart, fickle teenager that I was, but the memory of it still makes me cringe. We have all been there: it's 3 a.m., you can't sleep and you go over all the big moments of mortification that have happened in your life. Sometimes the cringe is so bad you make a little noise of embarrassment as the fear overtakes you. Luckily no one ever found out that I spent many an evening conversing with a hair-care product. Until now, I suppose.

One of the biggest issues I have had consistently throughout my life is sleep. More than any learning difficulty, disability or mental health problem, my sleep, or lack thereof, has had the biggest effect on me. I can go for days without even a minute of rest. On average, I get two or three hours' sleep a night. Five hours would be considered a triumph. I have tried every sleep aid, tip and method available to me. Nothing works. Falling asleep when you hear voices in your head is next to impossible. Never being comfortable when I am still stops me from sleeping too. It doesn't help that I hate the feeling of falling asleep, and that the thought of being unconscious for hours terrifies me. Though I don't hear voices in my dreams, I tend to have a lot of nightmares, and in general I will avoid sleep as much as possible while, at the same time, of course, craving the feeling a full night's rest brings. I don't go through periods of insomnia; it is a chronic thing and I can never recall a time when I slept well, even as a child. Going through life with little to no sleep has many physical and mental side effects. I don't remember a time when I did not feel tired.

Apart from self-injury and making myself sick, my other hobbies include obsessing over things. Not in the regular teenage-girl-falls-in-love-with-a-boy-band-member way, but in the obsessive compulsive, repetitive thoughts and compulsions kind of way. If I touch the arm of a chair, I have to touch the corresponding side in the same way, with the same pressure, for the same amount of time. I will keep going until I get it right, no matter how long it takes. I count everything around me, mainly steps, but other things too. I tap my fingers off each other, which has to be done a certain way or I won't relax until I am satisfied. Light-switch flicking, checking things are locked or turned off, all of these rituals must be completed. If I don't do them, I feel that something awful will happen to someone I love.

I must have messed one of my rituals up terribly, I think to myself, when Mam tells me she has cancer.

'I found a lump,' Mam says, as if it's nothing. 'I have to go for some tests.'

She has breast cancer. She says it's not as bad as it sounds. I don't know if I believe her. She has an operation to remove the lump. While this is going on I all but move into a friend's house and she does her best to distract me. I would love to tell you that I spend my days taking care of Mam and that I am a devoted, caring daughter, but the truth is I'm a bit shit when she is first diagnosed. I mind Gary as much as possible, but I can hardly stand being around Mam when she is sick. Age seventeen, I am at that incredibly selfish, egocentric stage of my life where I think the world revolves around me and my problems.

Mam goes for radiotherapy next. She winds up being the

first and only patient of Waterford's newest cancer clinic. My little Ford Fiesta sits in the middle of the empty car park while she gets her treatment once a week. I watch the construction workers as they build the remaining part of the hospital. You might think driving would be a major challenge when you hear voices in your head, but it is surprisingly grand. Most people listen to the radio in the car, it's the same thing. And the voices have a lot to say about Mam's situation.

'You gave her cancer. She's going to die. You'll have to watch the life drain out of her and that's what you deserve.'

Chapter 5

'We're in the money now, Freddie.'

I get my first proper job at seventeen in a restaurant. Not babysitting or helping out in the family shop but an actual real-life job.

Freddie: *We'll be loaded in no time, I'm sure. I'll be getting all the pussy.*

"Ew. You're actually disgusting. Did you know that?'

Freddie: *Thank you, I appreciate that.*

'You don't even have a body.'

Freddie: *Harsh reminder. I'm sick of boys, though, could you not experiment a bit?*

'No, we've been through this, I'm not interested in girls. You just have to get over it. Or you know, you could just fuck off altogether and leave me in peace.'

It's almost as though he pauses for dramatic effect, letting all the other voices in my head filter in.

'Get us out of here, you need to hurt. You're never good enough. If you would just listen, we can help you. Need to hurt. We need to escape. Find the cameras. Destroy them. They can hear what

you're thinking. Everyone is watching you. We're being followed.'

Freddie: *You going to get them to fuck off and all?*

I don't have a comeback.

I start in a week. One of my friends works at the restaurant too. The pay is decent, and since I am just starting to drive, it will help fund that.

It goes well, at first. Everyone is nice and it's an easy job. I do weekends and the time flies during peak hours. My friend and I work behind the bar, making drinks and desserts while being in charge of the takeaway orders.

Soon, though, I begin to have trouble with a man who is around the restaurant from time to time. It starts with staring, but eventually he gets comfortable enough to stop looking away when I catch him. He offers to take me home after my shift. His car is his pride and joy. 'I just want to show it off to you. Want you to see how fast it can go.' I turn him down every time, but he doesn't seem to get the hint. He is like this with most of the other girls, though, just an annoyance we have to tolerate. Creepy but harmless; that is how he is regularly described.

But this is not true.

It turns out that he has been taking photos of me on his phone. He proudly shows me his collection one day. I ask him to stop. He slaps me on the backside a couple of times. I ask him to stop. The staring continues, as do the suggestive comments, which get worse.

The following time he approaches me and says, 'I'll pay you.'

'What did you just say to me?'

'Young, pretty girls like nice things. I'll buy you whatever you want.'

I storm outside. I get a lecture from the head waitress for being dramatic. I am still hearing about how harmless he is from the others. He does this to all the girls, he means no harm, it's just his way.

His harassment gets progressively worse. I remind him, as I do every time he appears, that I have no interest in him. He is old enough to be my dad; actually, make that grandad.

No one in work seems concerned about what is going on. My parents would be furious with me if I got fired, adding to the list of my many failures in life. My mam has cancer and the last thing she needs is this, I tell myself.

One night, though, everything changes. I am standing in the car park at the back of the restaurant, having a cigarette.

I flick the ash and listen to Freddie talk as though we are the same person. He does that, thinks of himself like my weird disembodied twin.

What happens next is unexplainable. I get a profound sense of danger, my fight or flight kicking in without warning. I don't know how; it doesn't come from Freddie or any of the other voices, but something tells me I need to move fast.

Hide.

I slip in behind some parked cars, into the darkness. The man appears nearby; he must have just arrived at the restaurant. He lights a cigarette and looks up at the night sky.

Freddie: *Stay still. Don't even fucking breathe. He'll be gone soon.*

The man's head turns.

Please don't see me.

He comes over and I know it is serious. I play nice at first, trying to brush him off. He grabs me and pulls me to him. I haven't got a chance, I know there is no getting away.

Freddie: *We've been here before. We survived already. Even though you were much younger. Just try and get him off you.*

He's too strong. I give up after one pathetic attempt. I say no, I say stop, I say the things you are supposed to say but, after that, I freeze. In that moment, it feels like my body has completely betrayed me. There is no fight, no resistance, like my brain has lost the connection to my limbs and all I can do is try and escape with my mind instead. His slimy tongue licks my cheek over and over again. His hands are everywhere. I can't move, I can't breathe.

Freddie: *Think about something happy. It will all be over soon.*

There is a crash from inside the restaurant, someone has dropped some pots in the kitchen. Spooked, he gets off me and puts himself back together as he goes back inside. I am still frozen. My feet are rooted to the ground, my muscles seized up and there is still no air. A voice reminds me to breathe, to move; he could come back, I have to get back inside where there are people, where I will be safe.

Back inside the restaurant, I lock myself in a cubicle, rubbing my cheek where he was licking. I can still feel him, everywhere. Everyone is looking for me, the restaurant is busy, I need to get back to work. I shout that I will be out in a minute.

I open the cubicle and he is there, waiting for me. He

pulls me to him again, yanks my hair so I'm forced to look him in the eye. He searches my face, looking for something – fear, I think. Once he is satisfied that I'm scared enough, that I'm taking him seriously and not brushing him off as harmless like the other girls do, he takes my hand and puts something in it.

'You don't be talking.'

He lets go and walks down the empty hallway to the restaurant. I look at what he put into my hand. It's a fifty Euro note.

Once back on the restaurant floor, I ignore the lecture about taking too long a break. I don't know how I do it, but I somehow get through the rest of my shift.

Afterwards, I tell my friend straight away. She's horrified at first, encouraging me to report the incident. I can't see what I can report him for, though; he didn't get to finish, the noise from the kitchen scared him off, it doesn't seem serious enough to report. They will ask me why I didn't say anything sooner, how I could go back after my break and work, why I froze, why I didn't fight back. The freezing thing is what haunts me the most.

As a result, my friend's support does not last long. She thinks if it was serious or if I was upset enough, I would have reported it. She starts making jokes about it. She says I was stupid to smoke out the back of the restaurant alone. 'Do you not think you were asking for it?' Any thoughts I had of reporting the incident disappear. It was my fault. She is right, I was asking for it.

***

I live with the secret of what happened for a year. During that time, I get myself fired, intentionally; I don't like being around the restaurant any more. But I couldn't just quit; my parents would have been angry with me for leaving my first job without a reason. They are still pissed off when I am let go, but at least I can pretend it was somewhat out of my control. I cannot be selfish, putting this on Mam while she has cancer, but then, all of a sudden, the cancer goes away and she is in remission. The relief of being able to put that chapter behind us is incredible.

A few months pass and all I want to do is tell her. But I am afraid she is going to react like my friend did, so I hold off as long as I can.

'Selfish. Weak. It wasn't even that bad. Some people have it far worse than you. If you tell her she's going to get sick again and it will be all your fault. Blame. You're to blame for everything. All the bad things that happen, it's all because of you. Why do you have to be weak? We can make that better. Hurting yourself isn't weak. Only strong people can stand the pain. Listen to us and we'll make you strong. Stronger than your mother even. She can beat cancer, but can she hurt herself on purpose like you can?'

Finally, I wake her up in the middle of the night. I wait for her to chastise me for being stupid, for not saying anything, for freezing instead of pushing him away.

'I said all the right things. I told him to stop, I told him to get off me but I just froze then and let it happen. I only got away because someone dropped a pot in the kitchen next to us.'

I keep apologising until she cuts me off.

I get a hug. I hate hugs when I am upset, but my mother has always been the exception to the rule. She gives the best hugs, not the kind that make me feel smothered or trapped. They make me feel safe. It doesn't matter how old I get, I still look for them; they are the only hugs I ever seek out. She listens to me ramble more, whispering that it's okay, that everything will be alright.

When I have finally calmed down, I see her struggling, like she has something to say but is hesitating. I wait for her to ask me why I didn't report him straight away. That's not what it is, though; it's something else entirely.

'Do you mind if I tell you my story, about what happened to me?'

Mam grew up in Athlone. She was the oldest of three and she loved her two sisters, but she always felt like the odd one out in her family. She was closest to her father, she always said he was her best friend. He understood her in a way that no one else did. He died of cancer when she was thirteen. Nana was unable to work due to health problems and Mam felt she had to be responsible for far more than most young teenagers. She eventually dropped out of school to work full time. (Her lack of formal education was an insecurity of hers. She got upset when she couldn't help us with our homework, especially me, because I nearly always needed help.)

A year after her dad died, Mam took a babysitting job. The father of the children was a well-liked and respected man. And this man took a shine to her. He made dad jokes and she laughed. Sometimes his jokes bordered on being inappropriate, but Mam desperately needed the money and, in her naivety, she thought he was a harmless old fool. Until one day he attacked her at the back of the house. She froze too, she tells me. By the time she snapped out of her trance and ran away, he had done much more than the man had gotten to do to me. She went home to her grieving mother and said nothing.

The man also tried to attack the next girl who babysat for that family and word got out. Nana asked her if anything untoward had happened while she was working there and she said no. She says she didn't want to be selfish. The next girl didn't report him either. He got away with it and she never told anyone. Until now.

'There are men who are like that, Nicola, bad men. And they get away with it. Most of the time, people don't believe young girls. They want undeniable proof, which most of the time we don't have. It's wrong. It's unfair but life rarely is fair. It doesn't matter what we did or didn't do, those men did horrible things to us because that's what they are inside, we were just caught in the crossfire. We'll go after this man, if you want. But if it doesn't work out, if he gets away with it too, I want you to remember that no matter what anyone says, this was not your fault. It is never our fault.'

It is late or early, however you want to look at it. 5 a.m. to be exact, but there is one more thing. One more thing I want to say. I want to ask her is it okay if you let it happen more than once, is it still not your fault then? Is being young, really young and scared, ever an excuse for letting things happen and never saying anything?

'*Don't do it. You can't undo it. If you say it that will be it. You don't get to do this to us.*'

Freddie: *Do you really want to put that on her?*

Do you remember when I was really young and I used to say a man with no face came to see me sometimes? The words swim in my head but they won't come out of my mouth. They are stuck, permanently stuck. I let the memories sit there, broken and twisted. I can never remember all of it. I can't even recall what his face looked like. I made him up, just like I made up the bad woman.

I say nothing.

Chapter 6

During this same time in my life I meet someone who goes on to become quite important. A mutual friend introduces us. He says his name is Ishy. As in rhymes with fishy, sounds like squishy. I say that's hardly his real name, and he tells me that it's actually Kieran, and Ishy is just his nickname. He tells me the story behind the name and it's incredibly boring and uninteresting so I will spare you.

The next day I run into someone I know and Kieran/Ishy is standing beside her. 'This is my cousin. Have you met before?' she asks.

'Yes,' I say as he says 'No' at the same time. He gives me a confused look and I make a silent plea to the ground to swallow me up.

Freddie laughs.

Freddie: *Memorable as ever.*

Kieran and I become friends. I talk about boys with him and he talks about girls with me. He meets my family. Mam loves him, Gary looks up to him and for a long time I remain oblivious to what is really going on, even if everyone else can see it. In my defence, I am distracted with a few things. My Leaving Cert year has begun and I am incapable of studying. I have no idea what's going on in any of my classes and I feel just as lost as I was in first class when I couldn't hold a pencil. I still can't hold a pen right and I am eighteen years old. Everyone is talking about CAO points and where they are going to go next year. I know I have no chance at university. I gave up on the journalism dream when I realised I was too thick for anything academic.

Freddie: *So you're stupid. Poor Nicola, you know there's people with real problems? I can't take any more of you incessantly whining.*

The other voices have a lot more to say about my situation.

'You deserved what the man did to you behind the restaurant. Your mother is a liar. We can make it better. Turn off your phone, they can hear you. You don't need school. You're meant for much more than that. Everyone is watching. They are waiting. They put the microchip in your ear. You need to buy the salt; it will protect you from the witches. We are listening and we hear everything. We know what you have to do. Everyone is waiting, do you see them watching you? Don't look at the light. It's too bright for you. You have to kill. Make it bleed. Kill yourself and it will all be better. So much better.'

My thoughts have always been fast, racing through ideas, memories and plans faster than I could keep up, but they have sped up even more recently. It's the first thing I notice. Then the voices get louder. I feel a pressing sensation on my brain, like a fog that clouds my mind. When I wake up in the mornings there is a moment of calm, of nothingness. For that single minute I cling to the hope of this peaceful feeling lasting. But the voices flood in then and I am in what I call 'the bad place'. The bad place is where every happy memory is drained out of you and all you can see is darkness. The bad place is where there is no hope, you can't see beyond the next hour or the next day, there is nothing in the future for you, only this feeling.

'*Bitch. Useless. Why can't we go there? I like you. Horrible time of year. Fucking degenerate. Stop doing this to me. Worthless, worthless, worthless. He's coming for you. The world as we know it will end. You have to save her. Swim over here, you have to see it, it's beautiful. Do you think we could get a discount? Give up now. We found another way. He is trying to reach us; he can't get through. Why are you staring at it? Make me go away. Try to get there. Say your prayers now. I hate you. I hate everything about you. You make me bleed. I don't want you to be hurt any more. I wish you weren't here. You make everything bad in the world. They are listening. Warning. Danger. They can hear everything. Protect us. They are listening to us. Warning. Warning. They are here. They are coming.*'

Freddie: *You alright there, kid?*

'It's loud again.'

Freddie: *Oh no. Did you hear that?*

'Hear what?'

Freddie: *Listen, listen closely.*

'What? What is it Freddie?'

Freddie: *You can just about make it out.*

'You're scaring me.' I put my hands over my ears and shake my head.

Freddie: *I wasn't sure at first but it's definitely there.*

I don't reply, listening intently.

Freddie: *It's the sound of the smallest violin in the world, playing just for you.*

'Oh, fuck off,' I whine.

Getting up for school feels like climbing a mountain these days. I don't want to see people or talk to them; I don't want them to see me. I want to stay in bed, the safest place for me, with my earphones. Music drowns out the voices, the noise, the never-ending commotion that's eating away at my rational thoughts. The ones that I need to get on with my life, to be normal.

'Today is going to be a good day, Freddie.'

Freddie: *Sure, it is.*

Mam says I need to think positive thoughts. She's all into meditation and mindfulness. She's put these things around the house to block negative energies, there are crystals and angel cards, books on spirituality and well-being. Reiki, homeopathy, integrated angel therapy, she has taken to sending us to all this mad stuff where they try to solve all your problems by hypnotising you or sticking tiny needles into your skin. She claims it is what helped put her in remission. The high doses of radiation that they blasted through the cancer cells probably had a lot more to do with it, but whatever brings her happiness. My dad has worked in pharmaceuticals all his life, he is a man of science, so you can tell that it's difficult for him to agree that his hay fever is a result of his chakras not aligning properly. Still, he smiles and drinks his organic juice like the rest of us.

I do try the meditation thing in the mornings but it is hard to clear your mind when there are voices shouting at you. Instead I drag myself into school, late every morning. I have to sign a book and give a reason; 'I nearly bled out on my bedroom floor at four o'clock this morning' is not an excuse I can give without drawing attention to myself. The cuts are getting tougher to cover up, I keep running out of room on my skin to damage. I feel the pain of them all day, my arm throbs, I am lightheaded from blood loss and I have to keep changing the bandages so I don't get an infection. Sepsis is my main concern; I've learned exactly how to cut without going too deep or hitting an artery, but infection can happen at any moment if I am not careful enough.

HOW TO BE MENTAL TIP 6

Do not do any of the terrible self-destructive things I did to get out of the bad place. This does not get you out of the bad place, it just drives you deeper into it.

I count steps whenever I come across them: one, two, three, four, I count my own steps too. I count how many times I tap my fingers together and remind myself not to hold my breath in case I trigger a panic attack. I sit in class and try to keep my thoughts as neutral as possible. I don't know which of the people around me can hear my thoughts, but I am pretty sure it is all of them.

'Danger. Danger. We're in danger. Help us.'

There is no escape from them. They hear what I am thinking, they watch me. Everything I do, everybody is always watching. When I am at home there are bugs and cameras in my room and in my car too. I see cars following me all the time. I have to be safe, try to find somewhere safe where they can't get to me. I have to check my food too. There could be poison in there. I wouldn't mind dying but if the poison doesn't kill me it could make me sick or take over my body and control me, so I look out for signs, strange smells or packaging that looks like it has been tampered with. I don't eat if it's too risky, though on other days I eat and eat until I get sick. I've worked out that if cutting isn't enough there are other ways to hurt myself – I can make myself sick or bang my head against the wall. The little open sores I get on my hands from washing them too much hurt more when I dip them in bleach. I make myself sick when I feel sad too, as it releases some of the sickness inside me.

And I am sick. I know that much. I don't know what it is but something isn't right. I go from deliriously happy to sad and back again. When I am happy my thoughts race and the sky opens up shining colour on everything. No one can read my mind then, no one is out to get me, everyone loves me and I love them. I'm bursting with happiness, I don't understand how life can be hard, being alive is wonderful and I have the best life anyone could possibly have. I am the best person, I can do anything, my future is going to be the most amazing, incredible experience with endless possibilities. I can go anywhere, be anyone, the sky is the limit. The people around me are so nice, I like all of them and they can come with me and we will all live together in the big mansion I'm going to build. I have many ideas that are too good to not be successful, I will make millions. I have a new idea every minute, ideas that no one has ever thought of before. I can make everyone in the world as happy as me. I can cure cancer, solve world hunger, release all animals into the wild. I'll win a Nobel prize, all of them, an Oscar, a Grammy, I can win at everything. The world is beautiful, the colours around me shine so bright, the air is warm and the birds sing and nothing has ever been more perfect. I have never been more perfect.

But then the world slows down. Everything is dark. I remember every bad thing that has ever happened, every bad thing I have done. Everyone hates me and I am angry, no, furious at them all. There are too many problems: people are dying, they are sick and sad, they do awful things to each other, to animals, and I can't stop it. I am a terrible person. I do not deserve anything, nothing good will happen to me. I am guilty of causing bad things to happen to people, my mother got cancer because of me, it is my fault Stephen died, I've done such horrible things. And they are all watching me, they are coming for me. I need to hurt myself; I need to keep something sharp on me at all times, I need to keep cutting until there is no flesh left to cut. Get sick until all the badness inside of me is out. The demons that live in my mind are looking for my soul.

'Hurt. Hurt. Hate. Hate. Warning. We are all in danger.

Your fault. All your fault. Do you know why this happens to you? Because you're a bitch. Evil bitch. Drain the blood out from your wrists and make it all go away.'

Freddie: *Leaving Cert.*

'What?'

Freddie: *Your Leaving Cert exams. That's what you're supposed to be doing.*

I am in class. They are talking about how we need to knuckle down, we need to plan study sessions, practise mind mapping. The two teachers at the top of the room are saying things, more things. I know it's important, that I need to concentrate on it. Pre-exams, points, CAO, college, managing stress.

Freddie: *No stress. It's bad to stress, let's not do that.*

'They're listening. They are talking to you. We all know how thick you are. You can't do this. You won't do it. Other people go to college, they do their exams. You won't. Everyone is watching. Listening to your thoughts. It is not safe. Your thoughts aren't safe.'

I cannot study. I don't take in anything; I don't understand any of this. It's just words and numbers, none of them fit together. It doesn't make any sense.

Freddie: *You don't make any sense.*

'Why isn't anyone trying to help me, Freddie? Why can't they see something is wrong?'

Freddie: *I'm the only one trying to help you. But you can't tell anyone what you can hear. They'll lock you away. I know it's scary, I know it's getting worse. Don't tell them about us. Do you want to take pills that make me go away?*

'I want the others to go away.'

Freddie: *I'll get them away from you. I'm trying. I know this situation has gotten out of control. None of us meant for that to happen.*

Control. That's what I need. I don't have control over anything – except when I cut. It is the one thing that is mine. In school, they can have their good grades, their friends, their achievements, but none of them can do what I can do. They can't get a blade and put it into their skin, they can't twist it and drag it down their arm like I can. The voices go quiet. I have a head full of whispers. Something happens then. Something makes me angry or upset or frustrated. Then the shouting starts, louder, louder, louder.

'Someone's trying to kill you. Can you feel them? They are following you, watching you, you have to be safe. We'll keep you safe. There's a place where they can't get you. We'll take you there.'

I feel ill all the time. Not just in my head; I'm in pain. My stomach hurts, though I don't know if it's because I keep making myself sick. My left arm hurts, but on the inside, so I don't think it's from all the cutting.

Freddie: *Maybe you're dying.*

Dying. That's it. That's what I need to do, I need to die. I start to laugh, it's all clear to me now.

'Yes. Die. It's safe on the other side. We will all go together. No one will miss us here. Let's go. We'll go now. Over the bridge. Into the water.'

Freddie: *You're afraid of water. You can't swim.*

No, not water then.

'We will find another way then. Get in the car. Yes, that's it. Now put your foot on the accelerator. Push down. Don't look at the speed. Just keep going, push down harder. That's it. Nearly there, faster, faster, faster.'

Freddie: *Stop. Take it off, slow down. Come on, you'll end up killing someone.*

I slow down. Freddie is right, I can't do that to someone else.

I have these moments of clarity, where I am aware of time passing: days, weeks, months. I function surprisingly well from day to day. I can feel my mind slipping away from me, but the rest of me is on some sort of automatic mode. I am trying desperately to not draw attention to myself. At the same time all I want is for someone to notice, to help me.

I never really liked being alive all that much. I have been unhappy for most of my life. I don't know why exactly. I think it started with the faceless man or the bad woman. I don't know what made me make up these bad people. Maybe I was searching for an excuse or a reason for why I'm like this. I want more than anything to be normal. I want to be able to sit still, for my thoughts to slow down; I want the voices to stop, and I want to understand things in the same way that everyone else does. During these moments, where I can think clearly, I know that's never going to happen. I am never going to be normal. I don't know what I am but I know it isn't right. There is only one way out.

Freddie: *Your mother will be sad.*

'She'll get over it. She will forget about me. Everyone will.'

Freddie: *I thought we were going to move to Australia. You've got years ahead of you, kid; we'll do it all together. Just me and you. We'll shake the rest of these guys off and go live with the kangaroos.*

'I can't do it, Freddie.'

Freddie: *Stay a little longer. We'll figure something out.*

I hang on as long as I can. My brain feels like it is destroying itself. The voices are eating it up. I don't even care if I am going crazy or not, I'm just sad. I was supposed to grow out of this.

'Let's die. We'll all go together. It will be better. You're not good enough for this place. All the bad things you've done. We can't be here any more. You know here is not safe.'

I can't find the sleeping tablets. I am going to have to use the knife. I don't want to hang myself.

'Weak. Until the very last moment, you're weak. This is what you have to do. No backing out now.'

I find the pills. That is a relief. This is all about to end and I take comfort in that. I just want all of this to stop. I count out all the tablets. It is a bank holiday Sunday night; all my friends are out. My family are here, but they've gone to bed. No one will find me until tomorrow.

Freddie: *Please don't end us.*

I hesitate. What if I'm making a mistake?

'All the pain will stop.'

It plays out in front of me, all the hurt and pain, all the bad moments in my life so far.

'Fuck it.'

I take them all.

My phone rings. It's on silent. I watch the name flash up on the screen while I drift away.

'I wonder why Kieran is calling' is my last thought before it goes dark.

Chapter 7

Someone is shaking me. Slapping me. I hear my dad shouting my name. And Mam is yelling. I can see the morning light shining through the curtains. I hear my dad say there is no time for an ambulance. I black out again. It happens so quickly; it's almost violent how I am thrown into darkness.

Dark.

I am in the car covered by a blanket; I look up to the sky and hear my dad asking me to stay with him.

Dark.

I see my dad's car abandoned at the doors of A&E as I am carried into the building. I try to tell him he can't park there but am pulled down into the nothing again.

Dark.

I am surrounded by doctors and nurses. 'Waste of our time dealing with her. If they want to die, we should let them die.'

Dark.

'Why would you do this?' The doctor sounds angry. One of the other doctors is nicer to me. I cannot recall what she said but I know she is being kind.

Dark.

I am not in the emergency room any more but in a bed somewhere close by. There is a woman wailing in the corner, she sounds like she has just lost someone. Her screams remind me of the banshee I used to hear outside my window.

Dark.

My dad is sitting beside the bed. He is holding up my arm and a nurse is looking at it. Oh no, they know now what I have been doing. 'We'll get someone down to talk to her,' a doctor says.

Dark.

The fact that I am alive and survived the overdose is only really registering with me now. When I took it, I had wanted everything to stop, but here I am, alive, and I can hear the noise in my head. The shouting and screaming, all begging to be heard, all wanting me to listen, to pay them attention, and I don't even know why they are there. I need my phone.

Dark.

Fuck this. 'No, no, no, no. We don't want to do that now, do we?' a nurse says as she walks in on me ripping medical equipment out of my arms. She tuts. 'We'll have to put all of this back in again.'

Dark.

I get them all out this time and make it to the door, then down the hall, and stumble into the A&E waiting room. I see a room full of people look up at me in horror before I hit the ground.

Dark.

My dad is back and it looks like no one will be leaving me alone any time soon. Somewhere along the way I spoke to a friend and she is coming straight up to see me. At least she's not mad at me. My dad isn't either; he is just trying to understand what happened. My mam is furious, though; I remember her screaming angrily earlier.

I don't know how much time has passed. I am surprised to learn it's three o'clock in the day. I took the pills at midnight last night. I came here this morning but to me it feels as though only an hour or two have passed altogether.

I slip into the darkness less now. I am in a tiny room with big windows that look out to a busy corridor. There is a table between me and the man who has come to interview me. That is what they keep calling it as: an interview. He stares at me and I stare back at him. He has asked me why I tried to end my life and I said I wanted everything to stop. He then asked me to elaborate and we sat here in our staring contest ever since, which is interrupted by three security guards bursting through into the room. It turns out he pressed the panic button by mistake. After they leave, he begins firing questions at me.

Why did you do it? Had you been drinking? Have you taken any drugs recently? Are you stressed? Have you been feeling depressed? Any history of mental illness in the family? What is your relationship with your father like? Do you drink often? How many units do you drink in a week? Would you say you are a worrier? What about your diet? Do you think you're too fat or too skinny? When is the last time you ate something? How much do you eat on an average day? Have you ever been abused? Physically? Sexually? I can see the file he is writing in. There is a checklist and he's ticking boxes as he goes along.

We move onto the next phase; I can see a few questions together followed by a short paragraph space for him to fill in my answers. I tell him I hear noise in my mind.

'Do you hear it outside your ear or in your head?'

'In my head.'

'What kind of noise?'

'People talking, white noise, traffic sounds, running water, people shouting, singing.'

'Singing? Like a song.'

'Well, not like when you have a song stuck in your head, it's like that but it's different.'

'Everyone gets songs stuck in their head, it's when music we hear repeats in our head, usually something catchy.'

'Okay. I know that.'

Sometimes I get close to telling him about Freddie but then he moves onto the next question too quickly for me to describe the voices properly. He asks me what television programmes I watch; he asks me about the characters in the shows.

'Do you ever think you are those characters?'

'No.'

He gets impatient when I slur my words or struggle to get them out. I am still completely off my head and we have been discussing TV shows for far too long now. He asks me why I have been self-harming. I try to explain but I don't have a clear answer. He seems to expect me to tell him exactly what's wrong with me, but I was under the impression that was his job. I know he is a student; it says it on his hospital pass and he has brought some psychology books with him. I can't promise him I won't hurt myself again; he says he will have to sign me in as an inpatient in that case.

I'm tired and I am sick of talking. They don't have a bed for me that night so they send me home to wait. I go to bed with the door open. I wake up a few hours later and hear my parents whispering at the door. They don't want Gary to disturb me so they decide to close it. I am finally alone, as alone as I can be. I get my shoebox, full of blades, knives, bandages and a T-shirt soaked in blood. I have been waiting for this all day.

I don't want to go back to A&E. I just need to cut a little bit to get me through the night.

Slice. Slice. Slice.

***

The ward is small. There are a few single rooms, one of which I am in, and a bigger open ward across the hall. The reception desk is outside my room. My dad drops me off and stays for a while before going home. My mother cried when I left; she's not angry with me any more, just sad now. I don't want to upset anyone but it is too late for that.

A nurse helps me get settled in, she asks me why I am here and I tell her.

'But you're so beautiful, why would you do a thing like that to yourself?'

That is an odd thing to say, I think.

'We tried to tell you. We knew they would lock you up. No knives in here. You'll have to find something better. Couldn't even kill yourself right.'

I can smoke on the ward, which is most surprising. They light the cigarette for you at reception and then you sit at the circle of chairs and smoke.

I meet Darren here; he is addicted to heroin. He gets off it every few months, goes back to work as a delivery driver, gets sick in his head and goes back on the heroin and starts the cycle over again. He wants to cure his mental health problems before he ends up addicted and homeless again. He tells me how they wouldn't let him in here at first. He was in A&E when they told him there was nothing they could do to help him while he was still high. '"Fuck that," I said. "I'm getting in there. You have to help me," I said, "my brain is sick that's why I do the drugs in the first place." He laughed at me, started laughing in front of everyone at the front desk. Then they were all laughing at me. So, I said to him, "I'll be down in that ward by the end of the night." I started taking my clothes off. I started roaring then, said I was the devil and I was going to eat my own insides and rub them over the walls. I was grand, like, but it was the only way they would pay attention to me. I only got out to the car park and they came running up after me.' Darren spreads his arms out wide. 'And look where I am now.'

I get along with Darren the best.

Mary is another patient who frequents the smoking chairs. She is something of an escape artist. She got out only a few days ago – she made it to the taxi rank in her slippers and dressing gown. The taxi driver called the guards after dropping her off outside a shopping centre, so her adventure was short-lived.

There is an eight-year-old girl in the room next to me. I don't know her story and I don't think I want to know either. The nurses get sad when they talk about her. They are the nicest people here. One of them is my friend's mother. She freezes for the tiniest moment when she first sees me, before gathering herself; after that we pretend not to know each other. I meet another patient, Ben, and we discover we live near each other, around the same area. Ben takes to following me around. He asks for my exact address; I change it slightly. I don't think I want to be friends with him outside of here.

'Stuck in here now, you stupid bitch. No one is letting you out. We need to hurt. To bleed. Stupid, worthless, can't do anything right. I'll make things better. Just trust me. Don't listen to the rest of them. I'm the one that knows how to make it stop and I mean really stop.'

During my treatment, I am asked what I do when I get stressed, when my problems get too much. Saying that I cut myself sounds pathetic. Like I am too weak to cope with everyday life. I don't want to say it out loud. I raise my arm instead, which is bandaged, and gesture to it. I am asked more questions, too many, too fast. I keep my head down and whisper out short answers.

I am told that I have no signs of serious depression. I am told that I'm just stressed, my exams are coming. I am only eighteen years old and I am told that I probably never thought I'd end up in a place like this.

I did know. I think I have known for a very long time that this was exactly where I was headed.

I am told that harming yourself is serious, it is what people who are mentally unwell do. It is not something you do for attention.

I have nothing to say to that. I have been like this as long as I can remember. I have spent years hiding my problems, too afraid of what might happen if I told anyone. I hurt myself because it is the only thing I could ever do that gave me some kind of control. I make myself sick for that reason too. I have hidden the cuts and scars on my skin, cried in the cover of darkness, done all my suffering alone with no one to help me. I have finally asked for help and here I am, supposedly looking for attention.

One day, on the short walk back to my room, I pass Ben, who is on the phone.

'I have to go now,' he says to the person on the other end, 'Nicola is here.'

I bury myself under the sheets and go to sleep. It's the only escape I have in this place. They are watching me too closely for me to do anything and it looks like I won't be getting any help. I wake up to a pair of eyes staring back at me, an inch from my face.

It's Ben. 'You lied to me. You don't live where you said you live.'

He gestures to my hospital tag around my wrist with my

name and address on it. Someone comes in and pulls him out of the room before I can react. The next time I wake up, he's sitting in the corner of the room, smoking. The time after that he is sitting on my bed. Instead of dragging him out, they eventually put someone sitting outside my room to stop him coming in. No one says anything to me about it.

Darren leaves to go to the next ward. I don't know much about it; apparently it is less secure than this place. The main door here is locked shut and an alarm goes off whenever it is opened.

My mother comes to see me, I don't think I have ever seen her look so worried. She tries to get me to talk but I know it is pointless. I'm just a silly girl who wants attention, that's what the doctor said and that is what he will tell her. She gives up trying to understand and talks to me about normal stuff instead. Time goes slower than I ever could have imagined in here. I am relieved to be moved into the next ward.

Darren makes a big show of things when I walk into the smoking room there. He picks me up and twirls me around while all the new faces watch us. There are a lot more people in this bigger part of the hospital. I am the youngest here. Jenny, an American lady who is in the bed next to mine, takes to calling me baby. I don't have the heart to tell her there is an actual child in the other place. Jenny is the saddest person I have ever met; it is as though something sucked all the happiness out of her and all that's left is a shell of a person. She cries most of the time. Robert is in a wheelchair. He has scars all over his body, even on his head. One of the others ask him why. He tells us that he jumped out of a window.

'I ran straight at it. For a second, I thought I'd just hit the thing and bounce back onto the floor – that would have been embarrassing – but no, I remember going through it and flying through the air. It actually felt quite nice – before I hit the ground and broke nearly every bone in my body, that is.'

They talk about medication a lot in here: what dose they are on, the side effects. I am not on any medication; I have been told that even a mild antidepressant would be wasted on me.

'How are you finding the new dose?' a woman who has something called bipolar disorder asks another guy.

'It's alright. The side effects are more of a dose than any-thing. They make me thirsty all of the time and I can't stop pissing.'

'Are they doing anything for you?'

'Yes, actually, I have to say I feel well,' he says in his slow drawl.

'Really?' she asks.

'No,' he laughs.

Darren is annoyed because the doctors won't give him weed. He says it would be easier for him to stay away from hard drugs if he could just smoke it for medicinal purposes. He gets worked up and angry as he talks about it. He is paranoid and can't understand why they don't legalise it. He tells me things were better back when he just smoked weed on its own. Darren and I always sit with each other during mealtimes. He says we need to stick together.

'It's dangerous in a place like this.' I watch his hands shake as he reaches for the salt. 'We'll be alright, you and me, we have each other's backs.'

Freddie: *Okay buddy, we're not up in prison here.*

'Freddie!'

Freddie: *Miss me?*

'Where have you been?'

Freddie: *Around. I don't like us being here.*

'I needed you.'

Freddie: *I don't care if you needed me. You shouldn't have put us in here in the first place. I told you not to do anything stupid.*

'I just wanted it to stop.'

Freddie: *And has it?*

'No.'

Freddie: *You ain't getting rid of us any time soon, kid. At least you still have me, your favourite.*

'No, you're not. Anyway, I was supposed to die.'

Freddie: *Well, you fucked it. Now we have to sit in this shithole. I've got a plan to get us out of here, if we go to the doctor and say that you're feeling – oh hang on, Snoop Dogg here is trying to get your attention.*

'Are you listening to me?' Darren asks, waving his hand in my face.

'Sorry.'

'Where did you go? Your eyes went all spacey.'

I look at him for a moment and choose my next words carefully.

'I was listening to the voice in my head, we were having a conversation, inside my mind.'

Darren looks at me and nods. 'That's nice.' He goes back to telling me the benefits of weed.

***

A friend visits, laden down with magazines. I have been given my phone back and my clothes so I don't have to walk around in pyjamas any more. My friend has been great. She asks me too many questions, though, but I know she is just trying to understand what happened. She passes on the well wishes from our friends. My mam brings me a plastic plant and Jenny cries when she sees it. 'I wish someone would bring me a plant.' It must be lonely being in hospital in another country.

A lady comes to sit beside me on my bed. She introduces herself to me as the activities coordinator. 'Would you like to do some finger painting with us today, Nicola?'

Freddie: *Why is she talking to you like you're five?*

I decline.

My hay fever is acting up. The open window looking out onto the grass beside my bed probably isn't helping, but Jenny says she likes the fresh air and not a hope am I doing anything to set her off crying again. I have a pain in the sinus around my cheekbone, it only helps when I put pressure on it. Time is ticking along slowly and I have run out of things to do. I sit up, staring at the wall with a water bottle against my cheek to ease the pain. Two staff members enter the room.

'Hello there.' One of them waves. 'We're just here to change your sheets, we'll only be a minute and then you can go back to your, eh, your bottle.'

The other one laughs. As they change the sheets they talk as if I am not there. It seems one is new and is being trained into the job.

'Most of them are grand. If you talk slowly and don't make any sudden movements, they won't go for you.'

Trainee guy is too thick to realise the other one is only trying to scare him.

'Would they actually attack you?'

'Oh yeah, they bite the nurses and everything. Best part of the job is coming down to these wards, always something mental going on. Literally.'

They both turn to look at me.

'It's okay,' I say. 'The voices say I don't have to hurt you.'

Freddie laughs. The other guy even cracks a smile once he realises that I'm messing.

Freddie: *That was good. I like that.*

The doctors tell me that I am emotionally intelligent. I think they are trying to find a nice way of saying I'm thick but have a lot of feelings. I have given up trying to explain what is going on inside my head. I feel like they don't listen, they see what they want to see. At least they are not going on about how I don't belong in here, how the other patients are the ones with 'real' mental health problems.

'Life can be difficult for girls your age,' I am told. 'It is easy to get caught up in the … dramatics of things. We know you will be okay moving forward; we have every faith that you're going to be fine and you will be able to put all of this behind you. It isn't like there is any real mental health problem to hold you back, and that's what a diagnosis of depression would do, Nicola, hold you back,' they say.

There it is.

Freddie: *Showtime.*

I smile back at them.

Freddie: *Do you know what? I'm feeling much better. This place would put anyone in a good mood.*

'I'm actually feeling a lot better,' I say.

Freddie: *Excessively injuring oneself and taking copious amounts of sleeping tablets are the actions of a person with their sanity fully intact.*

'I know what I did was stupid.'

Freddie: *It's all thanks to you and your brilliant mind that I can go forth and leave this harrowing chapter behind. How foolish of me to think psychiatric inpatient care would be a fun time.*

'You're right, I don't belong in here. Seeing the other patients in here has really shown me how bad things can be.'

Freddie: *If you just sign off for me to be discharged, I'll just skip out of here. Thank you, from the bottom of my heart; thank you for your care and understanding.*

'I think I'm well enough to go home now.'

When I finish speaking, I make sure I smile with my eyes as well as my mouth. I learned that trick from practising in the mirror.

HOW TO BE MENTAL TIP 7

It takes a while to find a therapist that is right for you. Don't waste your time on one that is going to do more harm than good.

I say goodbye to Darren. I am sad for him; it is not his fault he's like this and I hope he gets the help he needs. I pack up my stuff as my parents wait for me at reception. Jenny says goodbye to me sadly before going into the toilet to cry, by the looks of it. I leave the little plastic plant on her bedside locker and all my magazines on her bed. As we walk out of the hospital, Mam stops to give me a hug.

'Things will be better now,' I tell her.

I have never felt more hopeless in my life.

Chapter 8

The initial few weeks following my hospital stay are weird. I feel as though I am under a microscope, everyone is watching me for signs of self-harm. I am not allowed near any sharp objects. The strangest thing is having everyone suddenly know secrets I have kept to myself for years. They may not know everything, but they know I have problems with my mental health, they know I have been hurting myself. It would make sense for me to drop the act now, but I quite literally cannot stop pretending.

Before I tell you this next part, I feel I need to explain things from what one of my friends once told me was their perspective of events: they have a best friend who, one day, seemingly out of nowhere, tries to kill herself. They expect me to act a certain way when I get out of hospital. I can't say how exactly they think I should be – sad, depressed, withdrawn would be my guess. I am none of those things, and this is where the problem lies. Here I am, behaving as though it's business as usual. They have never seen the side of me I keep hidden, the one that hears voices and believes all sorts of impossible things, the paranoid person who goes from delirious happiness to hopeless sorrow for no good reason. I have put on this mask for so long that I don't know how to take it off. I have been impersonating a normal person and now everyone knows that I am not, I am broken, and they want to know why. They want to know what happened to make me feel hopeless enough to end my life and I cannot give them a straightforward answer. Maybe it is because I don't have the vocabulary, or it's just too painful, or maybe it's because I have an illness that makes my mind go to such a scary place that there are no words in existence that could ever truly describe how it feels. And the reason I never told anyone? Why didn't I reach out and ask for help? After I was diagnosed with ADHD, nothing happened, there was no treatment. I simply had to carry on and learn how to function with this thing that lives inside my head and tortures me. There was never any mention of mental health, no one ever asked, so I didn't tell. Perhaps it's because of Freddie, but I have always had a dry, self-deprecating and dark sense of humour. I don't like to be the centre of attention or to be pitied. So, I make jokes, I brush off their sympathy because I don't know how else to handle the sudden attention.

I don't act the way they expect me to, I don't play the poor, sick victim role well enough and nothing could prepare me for their reaction. There are three of them in on it. They stop being my friends with no warning and no explanation. I notice more and more people being off with me. I am heartbroken to have my best friends up and leave me without warning and I don't understand what I have done wrong.

Our Leaving Cert exams start and I do mine in a room on my own with a supervisor (a trip to the psychiatric hospital gets you that sort of special treatment, apparently). I am also assigned a social worker with whom I meet once a week.

Kieran collects me after my last exam and we go and celebrate my disastrous school days being put behind me. This next bit is harder for me to talk about than my mental health problems, mainly because I am terrible when it comes to expressing my feelings. At this stage of my life I have had several boyfriends and none of them have worked out. I am not good at the romance thing, I have had two serious relationships and both ended when they said, 'I love you'. I responded to the first with 'Thank you' and to the second with, 'Okay.' I was a terrible girlfriend and they deserved better. But with Kieran it is different, I can just about manage to express affection without cringing and, after a surprisingly short amount of time, I even say my first ever 'I love you'. I am not quite sure exactly when I realised that we were more than friends, but as soon as I did, I just knew that he was it for me. Just three weeks after I leave the psychiatric hospital, we start a relationship that I know is for keeps; marriage, babies, the whole nine yards.

Freddie thinks it's hilarious at first.

Freddie: *Ishy. His name is ridiculous.*

'You're ridiculous and anyway it's a nickname.'

Freddie: *So, we're keeping this one around?*

'Yes, Freddie, we are.'

Freddie: *I can live with that, I suppose. Just warn me whenever I have to be present for the world's most awkward threesome.*

(Freddie is in my head most of the time and I can't get him out no matter what I'm doing. I know you were wondering.)

Kieran finds out why some of my friends have fallen out with me. He gets a phone call one afternoon, telling him how I'm a liar and an attention seeker. He gets a few more calls which go the same way. It turns out that they have been telling everyone that I was faking being sick. I cut myself for years in private, took an overdose and went to the psychiatric hospital for attention. This story spreads far and wide and I lose most of my friends because of it. Kieran is encouraged to break up with me, but thankfully he doesn't. I am going through one of the most difficult times of my life, while a group of people tell me they cannot wait to stand on the side-lines and laugh while Kieran and the remaining friends I have see me for who I really am and turn against me.

Years later, some of them did apologise. They said they didn't understand how I could be mentally ill but still act happy, making jokes and carrying on as normal. I told them that it was okay to not understand what I was going through, but there was no reason to be so cruel about it. Anyone with mental health problems will tell you the same thing – sometimes their suffering is as clear as day for anyone to see and sometimes it's hidden away. It does not mean we are faking being sick. I did, however, accept their apologies, and I am still close friends with one of them to this day.

With the others, it doesn't end there, it continues for many years, the turning people against me and generally making my life a misery. Having the type of paranoia I do, being afraid of people being out to get me is much harder when former friends are open about having it in for me. For years, one person in particular dominated a lot of my life and my mental health grew worse as a result. I could probably write an entire other book on the saga. Maybe they will read this book, expecting a detailed chapter on all the ways they seemed to me to try to break me. But I am only giving this person these few lines. I tried to muster up the anger to write about them but it's not in me any more.

> ### HOW TO BE MENTAL TIP 8
>
> When you live with hate in your heart, the only person you hurt is yourself. Projecting your pain onto someone else won't help to heal your own.

On the day of my Leaving Cert results I am surrounded by people celebrating their results: 400, 450, 500 points. They get enough to qualify for their dream courses. Someone is disappointed because they are five points off their choice and have to settle for second best.

Anyone with a mental health problem will tell you that sometimes the smallest of tasks can be overwhelming. The simple act of getting out of bed in the morning can seem impossible, basic self-care often goes out the window. It is not lazy, it is a loss of motivation, a recurring symptom found in almost every mental illness. To some people a victory might be completing a marathon or getting a promotion. For someone in the bad place, getting dressed is an achievement sometimes.

As you know, I found school challenging from day one. Two months after being discharged from the psychiatric hospital, I do my Leaving Cert. On results day, the first thing I do is ring Mam to tell her I have passed; she screams down the phone with happiness. I am delighted with my results; despite the odds, I passed. I am over the moon. I got 150 points.

HOW TO BE MENTAL TIP 9

Celebrate every victory, no matter how small. It may not seem like much to some people but you knew how hard it was going to be for you, yet you did it anyway. Be proud of yourself.

I study beauty therapy because that is what makes sense for me to do. I know I could do a PLC and get into journalism another way, but at the time I don't think I am capable of such a thing. I continue to see my social worker for a long time. I see a psychiatric professional as an outpatient. I sit in the waiting room with the other patients while we pretend not to listen to what is being said in the office. Whoever thought it was okay for a mental health clinic, where people go to talk about their most personal issues, to have paper-thin walls and a window on the door really didn't think that one through. Eventually I am put on mild antidepressants.

It's funny how the system works. If you go to your GP and tell them you're depressed, the best you can hope for is to get a prescription and to be put on a waiting list to see a psychiatrist. By the time the appointment rolls around, the season has changed, you have binge-watched several new series, your pregnant friend has given birth and you attended the christening last weekend; in other words, a significant amount of time has passed in your life. Your appointment might coincide with the best mood you have had in ages. On top of that, the appointment goes on for a maximum of fifteen minutes, but it is usually far less than that. They ask how you are doing and adjust your dosage of medication accordingly. You may get referred for counselling, which involves sitting on a waiting list for another long time, after which you get eight free hours of counselling and that's that. If you are still unwell, you can sit on another waiting list. I entered the mental health system with a bang when I had my suicide attempt, I skipped the GP referral part. Despite this, you can see how long it took me to even get on medication. This is the system the HSE has in place for people with mental health problems. People are being turned away at A&E because they are not 'sick enough' or there isn't a bed for them, only to go home and end their lives. People are dying of suicide every day. The system has failed; it does not work.

HOW TO BE MENTAL TIP 10

Try the system, be in the system but do not trust it completely. Have back-ups. Get on as many waiting lists as you can. Contact charities and organisations (there are many) that offer help. Ask a local TD to help you get appointments. If your GP tells you to come back if things get worse, then go back, even if that means turning around at the exit, walking back to reception and telling them it has, indeed, gotten worse and you're going to need to see the doctor again. You shouldn't have to fight to get help, it is not fair that you do, but you need to give yourself every possible chance to get better because you deserve it. Don't let anyone ever dismiss you, like I did, and waste years of your life being miserable because of one doctor's opinion.

I think this is the part of the story where the movies usually put the ending. Love cures all, the knight in shining armour sweeps me off my feet, we all live happily ever after. The end. Every movie that is supposed to raise awareness for mental health follows this formula. Character gets unwell, seeks treatment, leaves hospital a new person, meets someone, falls in love and it all works out. There is hope after all. They don't show you the after, they don't show you that mental illness is a lifelong situation.

HOW TO BE MENTAL TIP 11

There is no quick fix. If there was, everyone would do it. We would attend our short course of counselling sessions, pop some pills and everything would be better. God, I wish it was that easy. When you have mental health problems, the chances are you will have them for life. This is not to say the bad place has you forever, though. You will bounce between the good place and the middle place too. Some people are happy by default until something happens in their life to send them to the bad place, but people like us, we end up there for no reason most of the time.

The social worker doesn't do any special kind of therapy but he listens to me complain about all the trivial problems in my life while I leave out the scarier parts of my mind. I know it might seem ridiculous, wasting these sessions where I have someone's attention by talking about Kieran, friends and that fight I had with my mam over a hairdryer last week, but it makes sense to me at the time. These are normal problems for my age and I am a normal person. I am not one of the crazy people that get locked away in a padded cell. My normal problems are the same as everyone else's.

This is what I tell myself every day for the next two and a half years. I look back on photos of myself in those years and all I see is a happy girl who has a boyfriend and a family, even friends, lots of friends, which is something I had never thought possible – but there is a tribe for every kind of person, I suppose. I'm still studying beauty, passing all my exams and gathering lots of specialised qualifications. My life should be good but it is not and honestly at the time I don't know why. The link between hearing voices and severe mood swings never occurs to me. Maybe now is a good time to remind you that I am still at a place where I do not understand how it's possible for other people to not hear voices. They are the most normal thing in the world to me and even though I know there is something not right about what goes on in my head, I do not know any different. The voices' constant presence in my life is as familiar to me as breathing.

On top of that, I don't think people are listening to my thoughts or following me or spying on me. I don't think they are; I know they are. To me it is all real. And it is making me angry. I am pissed off at everyone in my life for not being honest with me. Why are they lying? Why don't they just admit they are watching me? I'm never alone, I always get the sense that there is someone lurking in the shadows, possibly invisible, and they are all waiting for an opportunity to hurt me.

Sometimes I can push it all into the back of my mind, put a smile on my face and the world doesn't know I am breaking. Then it gets bad again and I am consumed with thoughts of hidden recording devices and telepathy. And sometimes, leaving all strange beliefs and disembodied voices aside, I am just really fucking sad. There doesn't have to be a reason most of the time; this darkness comes over me and I sit in the bad place and feel the emotions that live there: misery, hopelessness, despair.

I want to pull myself together and be happy; after all, isn't that what everyone wants? But when I think about the positives in my life, I feel guilty for being sad when others have it much worse. When I think about the future, it scares me. The past haunts me and the present is too overwhelming.

Then the euphoria comes and I am the happiest I have ever been. It lasts a few hours at most, my mood going up and up, but the higher it goes, the worse the crash back down is.

It is only a matter of time before things fall apart again.

Chapter 9

My breakdown happens much quicker this time. I have been spiralling for weeks (or has it been months? I don't even know myself) and it all blows up one night. It is more dramatic and more public than my previous episode.

Kieran and I go back to one of our friends' houses after a night out. It is not even the alcohol that does it, but something in my mind snaps. After twenty years of silence, I turn to Kieran and say, 'I can hear voices in my head'. The floodgates are open then, the walls come crumbling down and my big secret is out; I try telling him everything all at once. I get angry and frustrated when he won't listen properly. I need him to move past his confusion and listen to what I am trying to tell him. If I tell him about the voices, I've decided, he can explain to me why he ever agreed to be in on the 'big plan' to go to Australia. He is supposed to love me more than anyone, but he is like the rest of them. They all watch me, and talk about me, and read my mind, and I want to know why he joined them instead of sticking up for me and telling them all to leave me alone.

It's not working, he's not listening. On to the next one then. I tell my friend and he doesn't believe me either. But of course he would say that, he can't ruin the plan; after all, I could be bluffing about figuring it all out. I tell another friend; he pretends to be confused too and they are all liars and I need to talk to someone I can trust. The voices in my head are screaming, roaring at me so that I can't even hear what they are saying. There is no sign of Freddie and I need him to tell me what to do next.

Sylvia. My aunt Sylvia won't lie to me, I will tell her. If Sylvia is annoyed to be woken in the middle of the night, she doesn't let on. I sit on the stairs of my friend's house and tell her all the bad things that have been going on. I am not sure if she has been in on it; it's too hard to tell over the phone. She is going to tell my parents so I don't have to, which might not be the best idea because it will give them far too much time to come up with a story. I don't want to believe in any of their lies any more. Kieran, my family, my friends have all been lying to me and pretending to love me; they are all in on it and I want to know why they are doing this to me.

I go into the toilet and can hear Kieran talking to my friend in the next room, worrying over what to do with me.

After I have cut my wrists, I let the blood run for a while until my head spins. I walk into the room, in all my bloody and crazy glory, and say, quite casually, 'You're not supposed to leave me on my own.'

***

Mam takes this incident better than the last one. All her research on mental health and 'How do I help my depressed daughter?' googling saw to that. She brings me to A&E, where I explain as much as I can to a nurse. That he looks wary of me is the first thing I notice. No one has ever looked at me as if they have a reason to be cautious before today day. 'I need my mam,' I announce suddenly when I feel I cannot cope without someone who knows me being by my side.

This nurse escorts me to the psychiatric ward. Mam goes off to talk to someone after that and another nurse brings me to an empty area and pulls a curtain around us. 'Why would you do a thing like this?' she says angrily as she tends to my wounds. Cutting myself has remained an on-and-off habit these last few years. I would do it all the time if I could get away with it, but Kieran and Mam check me for cuts regularly.

The nurse leaves and I stand in my allocated little area and wonder what happens next. Suddenly someone grabs me from behind and stabs me in the back with something. It's the nurse; she came back and gave me an injection and literally ran away straight after. When she comes back, I tell her I am not afraid of needles and she could have warned me, it wouldn't have been a problem. 'Some people can react badly to the idea,' she says. Oh. It's like that then.

Freddie: *Ha. She thought you were going to hurt her.*

'Where have you been?'

Freddie: *I leave you alone for five minutes and you ruin your life.*

'What was in that injection anyway?' I ask the nurse.

She tells me it was a tetanus shot. She starts running through questions on her clipboard, the same as the last nurse asked me.

'Are you hearing voices right now?'

'Yes'.

Freddie: *Cunt.*

'What are they saying?'

'This and that.'

I am put in the same room as last time with the big window. I sit across from a student with his questions and answers book on the table. We run through them, same as last time, only I am not high from an overdose and can answer with more clarity. I tell him about the voices and all the things I believe to be true at the time. When we finish, he says to expect a letter to attend the clinic in the post soon. I will wait weeks for it and the appointment will be several weeks after that, if I am lucky. I complain to Mam about this on the way home. She tells me not to worry, we'll go private and hope the health insurance covers most of it. 'I'll find somewhere,' she says 'and if that doesn't work, we will try somewhere else. We will keep trying until you're better.'

***

There are two people assessing me at the private clinic: Kate and Julie. I see Kate first. I am not sure of their official roles, but Kate is the one who does the talk about your problems and Julie is the one who tells you what is wrong with you and gives you medication. We move through the usual checklist quite quickly. Kate is a nice person, and she is good at her job, but I imagine asking people the same questions repeatedly can get a little mundane after a while. She has her sympathetic face on and is using her soft voice, but when I listen closely, I think I can detect the slightest hint of boredom.

When she gets to the 'Are you a worrier?' question, I nod and she asks me what kind of things worry me. I tell her voices in my head are usually at the top of my list of concerns. You have probably guessed that we are getting close to the point of the story where I get diagnosed with schizophrenia. Over the next eight years I will sit in front of many new mental health professionals, whether it be because I have been referred for a different treatment or because the last therapist wanted rid of me. No matter how unwell I am or how tiring it gets filling in yet another person on my mental health history, the look on their face when they realise that they are dealing with psychosis never gets old. Well, two looks: there is Category 1, this is going to be a great challenge, and Category 2, oh shit I didn't sign up for this.

I have Kate's full attention, then, as she asks more in-depth questions, hanging on my every word, which seems a little unfair for people who come here with depression, but I suppose the less common an illness the more concern it gets. She asks the same questions they always ask. I answer as honestly as I can. I tell her about the voices, the mind reading, the people who are watching me, following me, how I am never alone. She asks me why I am tapping my fingers off each other. I tell her I have to do it or something bad will happen. She asks if

I have any other quirks. I tell her how I can't stop washing my hands, how I need to repeat things a certain way or in a specific order so I don't start some kind of butterfly effect where a catastrophic disaster will occur. She asks me do I have any questions for her. 'Can you do something for me? Can you make me normal? Like all the other girls my age, can you make me like them?' I know I am wide-eyed; my leg is shaking uncontrollably; I'm twitching a bit and my tone of voice is frantic. I haven't slept in days. I don't feel real; this seems like I am in a dream.

We go to see Julie next and I learn that Julie loves drugs. She prescribes lots of medication for me. I hear words like psychosis, bipolar, schizoaffective disorder. This is the first time anyone has ever said those words in relation to me. She talks about a place I can go for assessment, a hospital I can go to where my condition can be observed. They have treatments there for people like me. They might be able to help.

Schizoaffective disorder – it is not an official diagnosis, yet, but I know it is inevitable. It feels like a sentence. I always knew there was something wrong with me, but this is too much. I am full-on, properly mental. It wasn't supposed to be like this, I was meant to grow out of all of it. I was a weird child who would grow up and be magically better. Would I ever be allowed a visa for Australia? Can people with the word schizo in their diagnosis even work? Will I be allowed to have children, what if I pass it on to them?

I take to my bed for days and torment myself with these questions. I look at the generic information on psychosis online – signs, symptoms, treatment, recovery – but there isn't much detail. I watch a documentary on YouTube from the 1980s about schizophrenia where the contributors describe how the voices tell them to kill people while the voiceover talks about the madness that lives amongst us. I know now that the entire thing is pure sensationalism, an attempt to increase viewings, but when I first watched it I was terrified. I don't want to hurt anyone; I have never had a homicidal thought in my life. Is Freddie going to one day demand that I off someone? Freddie can be awful; he says appalling things about people sometimes, but he never suggests anything violent. The bad voices only ever suggested I hurt myself, never anyone else. I search the internet relentlessly for personal stories of the illness. I am a lot more successful when it comes to bipolar disorder but cannot find anything on psychosis or schizophrenia that makes me feel positive.

There is a small sense of relief in knowing what might actually be wrong with me after all this time. Psychosis affects your thoughts, feelings and behaviour; it can impair them to a point where it decreases your ability to understand reality. There are several psychotic illnesses. Schizophrenia has two types of symptoms – positive and negative – but keep in mind, these words do not have the typical, happy/sad, good/bad meaning here. Positive symptoms are auditory hallucinations or voices you hear in your head (hello, Freddie), and visual hallucinations like the things I used to see when I was a child, such as pictures moving, people, etc. Tactile hallucinations create a feeling of things moving on your body, like rats or insects crawling up your legs. Smells can also be hallucinated. Other positive symptoms are disorganised speech (stuttering over words, sentences not coming out properly), trouble concentrating, and problems with movement. One of the main positive symptoms is delusions – the false beliefs or paranoid thoughts I can have. Negative symptoms include difficulty expressing emotion (shout-out to *Big Brother* for help on that one), social withdrawal and struggling with basic daily life and finishing tasks. Meanwhile bipolar disorder, which was once called manic depression, causes unusual or extreme shifts in mood, energy and activity levels. It also causes hysterically happy moods along with exceedingly low periods. The different types of the disorder – Type I, Type II and Cyclothymic – are usually defined by the severity of the episodes (the period of time a manic episode lasts for) and how severe the mania is (hypomania is less severe), along with many more factors. Manic episodes can increase activity levels and cause rapid, racing thoughts, reckless behaviour, poor decision-making, increased self-esteem or unrealistic beliefs in one's abilities, over-excitement, irritability and frustration. A low mood is a deep depression. Schizoaffective disorder is a combination of schizophrenia and bipolar disorder, which is what I am suspected of having.

My new medication means that I cannot drink alcohol any more, which may not sound like a big deal, but when you are twenty-two it really is – at least to me. I feel like more of a freak than I ever have before. And that's not the only issue with the medication. Most people on anti-psychotics, when they list out all the horrible side effects, will start with the most obvious one: weight gain. You know in *Mean Girls* when Lindsay Lohan gives Rachel McAdams those bars that make her put on weight really quickly? Well, anti-psychotics are a bit like that. They also make you feel like complete and utter shit, as I soon learn. We fiddle around with the medication quite a lot, trying to get the right dosage with the least side effects. They put me on tablets for anxiety too, which seems like a good idea to me.

Anxiety is more like a symptom of schizoaffective than anything else, but I am learning enough about it to know it is a condition that definitely applies to me. There is a big difference between worrying about things and actual anxiety. Most of us panic when it comes to public speaking, starting a new job or meeting new people, but the fear passes once the threat is gone. Real anxiety means the threat always feels like it's there, even when it's not. It doesn't have an off switch. Real anxiety causes you constant worry, avoidance, insomnia, stomach issues and panic attacks. It is much more than being nervous.

Back when I was in hospital for the overdose, Gary had wanted to know if I was sick. Mam told him I was and when he asked where I was hurting, she said 'in her head'. One day, while I am lying on the couch questioning my existence, Gary throws a blanket over me. He tells me he heard I was sick in the head again and asks if I want to watch his *Inbetweeners* box set with him.

HOW TO BE MENTAL TIP 12

It's okay to talk to children about mental health. They understand it better than us sometimes.

This is how I spend my free time outside of college over the following weeks, with Gary and Kieran, on the couch watching mindless television until Mam occasionally gets tired of watching me mope and drags me out to do something somewhat productive. I moan and complain that I don't want to do anything – I am sick, after all – but she won't listen.

Mam has this rule. You must only allow yourself to be sad about your problems for a certain allocated time every day. When that time is up, you have to block it out of your mind until your 'sad time' the next day. Mam has been forcing this life lesson on me since Stephen died.

Every day she wears her best clothes; hair blow-dried and a full face of make-up. I can count how many times I have seen the woman in a tracksuit or with her hair tied up. She has always been determined to look her best, as though looking good on the outside somehow made everything on the inside okay, and she is forever trying to get me to do the same.

'That's easy for you to say, you don't have a mental illness. I can't apply your stupid rule to my life because there is something wrong with me that forces me to be sad no matter what I do. It isn't fair,' I would whine at her every time she tried to drag me out the door, until one day she snapped, 'You're right,

I don't have a mental illness but I lost my father, I lost my child and then I got cancer. Life isn't fair.'

She has a point.

Once I finish my exams, I get ready to go to the psychiatric hospital again. I know I am incredibly lucky and privileged to go into private care. I hope this works; I really do.

Chapter 10

My first few days as a psychiatric patient in a secure mental health facility for the second time are mostly consumed with thoughts of Jedward, the twins from *The X Factor* with the big hair. Without context, that may seem peculiar.

This particular hospital works differently from the stereotypical mental health hospitals you may have seen in the movies. It is not even like the one I was in before. Patients have a lot more freedom here. If you are not considered to be at risk of self-injury or suicide, you can basically go anywhere as long as it doesn't interrupt your treatment. All you need is to pick up a pass at reception and off you go. You can go shopping, to the park, run errands, meet a friend, whatever your heart desires, as long as it doesn't clash with your scheduled treatment times. You even get to go home at the weekends.

I, however, am at risk of self-injury and suicide, so I have to spend my first few days, which happen to fall on the weekend, in the hospital with a small handful of other patients who are not weekend-trip-home-approved either. Nothing happens at weekends, as the place is mostly empty. Just a few of us sad sacks are wandering around or watching the TV in the smoking room. Since we are all bored beyond belief, both we and the staff spend that first weekend immersed in *The Eurovision Song Contest* where Jedward are competing with 'Lipstick'. Somewhere between Denmark and Lithuania I get introduced to everyone. I am alarmed when one of the patients tells me they have been a patient here for years. I am even more alarmed when they tell me their diagnosis is schizophrenia.

You get surprisingly used to a lot of things while in institutional care, but the slow passage of time is never one of them. It is only two days but it feels like we spend an eternity listening to Marty Whelan and watching people parade around the stage, all feathers and fabulousness. The rest of my fellow patients arrive back on the Sunday evening and the ward looks like an arrivals lounge in an airport. The younger patients act as though they are rocking back up to their student accommodation for another week of college after going home to get some clothes washed and a few good dinners from their mammies. Being the newbie is never fun, but I make friends quickly.

The hospital is a huge building. It has several wards, a garden, library, gym, chapel, an art room, other various activity rooms and different departments for cognitive behavioural therapy, occupational therapy and so on. I see the main doctor once a week. Every few days, I announce that a terrible mistake has been made and I don't belong here. I want to go home. There has to be an easier way than this.

There are different activities going on every day. You can go to a drama class, make jewellery, attend art classes, learn pottery making, go to movie club; you can work out in the gym, pray in the church if you are that way inclined, or attend talks. One day, randomly enough, Christy Moore comes in for a performance. On paper, it probably seems like a spa retreat, but after the first few weeks you grow tired of all that; after a couple of months, it becomes plain monotonous.

When you are struggling severely with your mental health, looking ahead is difficult. As someone who likes to have a plan, I like to look ahead and foresee what I imagine my life to be like in six months, a year, three years. My mental illness undermines this. I can wake up with relatively calm thoughts, only to end up in a fit of paranoia and anxiety by the time I have showered and dressed. My mood, my outlook, my emotional state changes by the hour. I cannot look ahead to the next time I see the head doctor, or when Kieran is coming to visit, or when I get to go home for a weekend, because, in here, two hours feels like two weeks, and when my mind is in the bad place, I cannot imagine how I can withstand another minute. But I do. I live in the moment, hour by hour, and wait. Wait to feel better, wait for something to happen that will take me out of the bad place.

Every morning, instead of thinking about the almost empty fifteen hours that lie ahead until I can crawl back into bed again, I attend my psychosis programme. There are only a few of us on it. Every day we sit in a circle with a different mental health professional, be it a psychiatrist, a nurse, a social worker, a psychologist or a pharmacist, and we learn about recovery strategies, life skills, medication, cognitive behavioural therapy (CBT), future planning and social skills. I am not sure if it is actually doing much good, but at least it means I have a time and place where I am expected to be, a routine. Most stuff is optional, but I am trying to earn a few brownie points with the staff, come across as a model patient throwing herself into her recovery. The more they trust me, the more freedom I can get.

I am not permitted to go out alone. Sylvia visits once a week and signs me out for a bit. Mam comes to see me almost every day. She gets a lecture from the nurses about her mollycoddling on more than one occasion. It doesn't matter that I am over a hundred miles from home, she knows I need her. She has told me many times that she doesn't understand any of it: psychosis, hearing voices, anxiety, feeling depressed or hyper, but she is there for me and, even though none of it makes sense to her, she treats me the same way she would if I were in hospital for a physical illness. Even when Dublin practically shuts down because Queen Elizabeth is making a state visit, Mam makes it in to see me. She does the same when the president of the United States, Barack Obama, comes to Ireland a week later. It was an eventful summer for Ireland.

I talk on the phone to Kieran every night and live for his visits. One day, he only has a short window available with work so he makes a six-hour round trip to see me for just half an hour.

In the psychosis programme, we try to understand what caused our psychosis, which is my cue to sink into my chair and hope I disappear. In a one-to-one session, we talk about how my hallucinations began and about the moving pictures. But mainly the focus is on people I used to see, the faceless man and the bad woman. I still see pictures or photographs move occasionally, but I don't see those people any more.

In one of my first assessments at the hospital, a junior doctor is looking over my file. She is nice, a bit soft, and the other patients mock her a lot because she has a funny name, but I like her. 'Can I ask you something? There is a man that you have mentioned a few times now, one of the visual hallucinations.' I nod. I can see where she is going with this and I'm not sure I like it. 'Is there any chance that this man is real?'

Freddie: *Whoop there it is.*

I want to give her the honest answer. The truth is, I don't know. I imagined a lot of things when I was little. But he was different. He wasn't like the others; he could touch me.

Freddie: *You and I both know the truth. Just say it.*

'No,' I answer. 'Absolutely not.'

Freddie tells me what I should and shouldn't say. He tells me to leave out anything about making myself get sick because if I don't, they will move me to the wing for eating disorders and I don't have one of those. I have seen those girls and I look nothing like them, I clearly don't belong there. Freddie also says that I shouldn't tell them about him and I agree. It's one thing having lots of random voices who say pointless, meaningless things, but trying to get them to understand that there is one particular voice who is present all the time and has an actual influence on my decisions makes it sound more

SANE

serious. I want the voices gone, as I know my life would be so much better if I was normal, but I am having a hard time contemplating the idea of not having Freddie around. I try to have that thought as silently as possible so he doesn't hear it.

HOW TO BE MENTAL TIP 13

No matter how many mental health problems you might face, you cannot deny having any of them. They are not a selection of pick and mix where you get a choice on which ones deserve to be treated. Not getting help for all your issues is only going to delay your overall recovery.

They put me on more medication on top of what I was already on when I got here. Anti-psychotics, antidepressants, anti-anxiety, Valium, mood stabilisers, sleeping tablets. More get added with every week that goes by. The side effects are horrendous. The anti-psychotics cause me to rapidly gain weight; I have vivid nightmares; I feel dizzy and nauseous. My speech is slurred and my vision blurry. I have trouble focusing on anything and my peripheral vision goes. My hands shake and I can't manage even a minute of sitting still, eventually developing restless leg syndrome (RLS). Then the pain starts. I can feel it deep in my bones; my joints are stiff and it hurts when I move. I am stuck in an endless loop of trying to stop my legs moving as it is hurting me, but as soon as I get them to stop, the uncomfortable sensation of RLS becomes too much to bear and I start the torturous cycle again.

There is a mix-up with my medication one week. I am taken off a tablet which, it turns out, is actually quite important. It starts slowly. I get a strange out-of-body experience a couple of times, which I say nothing about because I don't want to add it on to the ever-growing list of my problems. The sensation lasts for just a moment at first, but the next day it goes on for an hour. A day later, it's like something in my mind breaks. I feel a cord that connects me to everything in my life – Kieran, my friends and family, Freddie, my conscious thoughts – and the cord just snaps. I don't know who I am, they keep calling me Nicola, but I don't know who that is. I know I need to drink water to survive, so I keep drinking it. Then I need to pee. I keep going from downing water to using the toilet and back to repeat the process again. If I need food, I'm going to have to hunt for it and I'm not sure where I would find animals in a place like this. The walls are in my way, I can't walk through them so I keep rubbing them. They feel strange. Everything feels strange, different. The colours are different too; everything is so bright and loud. Sounds have colours and colours have sounds. I can feel the skin on my body, I can feel my organs, no I can hear them, working away inside me. I need to make sure they don't stop; I must find a way to stay alive. If I can get through these walls, I can find something to hunt.

I don't remember much of what was going on around me at the time, but apparently I caused quite the scene. Eventually a medical doctor is called to see me and she works out the source of the problem. The reason I am acting like Bear Grylls on an acid trip is down to my medication. Now, I cannot for the life of me remember the correct medical or pharmaceutical terms here, so I am just going to explain it as best I can. I was taken off a pill that contained a chemical which I am going to call 'Juice'. Now this Juice had the job of counteracting the more serious side effects of my anti-psychotic medication, of which I was on have been prescribed the maximum dosage. A student doctor (let's not judge him; it's like how you should respect learner drivers – we all have to start somewhere) signed for me to be taken off Juice. It took a while for the drug to fully leave my system, and as it did I had those few odd out-of-body experiences. But when all the Juice was gone, I ended up having that episode. So the doctor gives me an injection of Juice, and over the next week or so I am given high volumes of it so I can build up the correct amount of it in my system again. While this is going on, I have a few more of these incidents. Of all the bad mental health experiences I have had, I can honestly say that was the worst.

Temporary trips down insanity lane aside, I seem to be doing somewhat okay. Every now and again a discharge date is mentioned as a possibility, but then I get bad again and end up back where I started. I notice I am not the only one who follows that pattern. Someone on the ward can be in great spirits, talking about their plans for when they get out and looking forward to the future. In the space of a day or even a few hours it all changes and they are in a bad way again. Some people actually get to leave, only to appear again weeks later. I am learning that while recovery is hard, staying well is where the real challenge lies. Talking to patients who have spent their whole lives in and out of hospital scares me. That's not the life I want, but I suppose that's not the life they wanted for themselves either. Mental illness is not a choice. There is not a single person in this hospital who would choose this over being on the outside, coping well and getting on with life.

Part of my treatment is a young adult programme where we have group sessions. It is a recurring trend that most of the others have someone in their lives; a parent, a friend or a partner, who think they are throwing their life away. Myself included; I know some people think I could just snap out of it if I wanted to.

On my weekend trips home, I cannot drive any more because of the vision problems. My slurred speech and slowed movements make me look drunk and I have heard that this is amusing to some people. That hurts. I wish you could see psychosis. I wish I could show the people in my life who don't understand what it's like to be trapped inside a mind that is broken. If they could just experience it, even for a minute, they might go easier on me.

How I ever thought people could read my thoughts is beyond me. The logical part of my brain has finally taken over and I can see how my delusions are part of my illness. Every time I start to get paranoid thoughts, I think: 'It's not real, it's just because you are sick right now'. It takes hours or even days sometimes, but I am getting better at it. This is what diagnosing, or that word that I hate so much – 'labelling' – does. It gives you knowledge and knowledge gives you the power to take some control of your condition.

Speaking of knowledge, I learn many new things about the mental health spectrum during my time at the hospital. Did you know there are over 200 classified forms of mental illness? Depression and anxiety are the most common. Most of the people on my ward have obsessive compulsive disorder (OCD), which has far less to do with cleaning than you would think. Some people have the fear-of-germs type that most of us associate with OCD, but I only meet one person like this. He cannot touch anything without using gloves or covering his hands with his sleeves. And when I say anything, I mean anything; even the simplest tasks, like using a door handle, are distressing for him. He stays in bed most of the time.

OCD goes far beyond being a clean freak, though; it is an anxiety disorder which causes unwanted images and intrusive thoughts. These repetitive thoughts or images are called obsessions; they can come in many forms, as can 'compulsions', which are acts people with OCD typically use to try to rid themselves of their obsessions. (A compulsion can be anything from turning a light switch on and off to counting up to a certain number.) Just to be clear, no one with OCD chooses their obsessions. They are extremely frightening and can lead to the sufferer feeling ashamed. I meet one man who is scared he is going to harm a child. He has never had any desire whatsoever to hurt anyone, never mind a child, but his illness tricks him into being scared that he is going to lose control and randomly carry out this act. Have you ever been talking to someone and just thought: *imagine if I just suddenly punched them in the face?* Or have you ever been standing near water and had this weird little fear that you were suddenly going to throw your phone or yourself into it for no reason? There are little niggles, quirks and random things that pop into our heads that are totally common because our brains are weird and they like to play tricks on us. But with OCD these thoughts are constant and completely out of control. A person with OCD usually knows that their obsessions are unrealistic, but they cannot ignore them. These obsessions can completely take over a person's life, causing them severe distress. Those with OCD usually employ compulsions as a sort of coping mechanism to deal with their obsessions. They can temporarily reduce the anxiety or fear, but the more the compulsion is carried out, the stronger the urge becomes to continue using this response to an obsession. Compulsions can also occur on their own, separate from an obsession.

Through the other patients, I also learn about borderline personality disorder (BPD), an illness that causes abnormal patterns of behaviour and mood, extreme emotions, distorted self-image and view of others, as well as difficulty maintaining close relationships. BPD also comes with intense feelings of abandonment and fear of being alone. It has many symptoms – impulsivity, risk taking, antagonistic behaviour, difficulty controlling emotions, feelings of neglect or being misunderstood. BPD is often missed or overlooked when searching for a diagnosis. It does not make someone a bad person, but it does make their personality confusing – not just to everyone else, but also for themselves. Feeling like you want to be alone but at the same time craving company, fearing rejection, illogically analysing everything; surely most of us can relate to those?

However, with BPD these feelings and behaviours are not only extremely intense but can also, at times, be completely out of control. People with BPD feel emotions far more intensely than a neurotypical person, but they also love deeply too.

They say you are not supposed to make friends here (in case we influence each other and make our issues worse), but it is almost impossible to live in these conditions and not become close. Any employer who wants their employees to bond should just throw them into a makeshift psychiatric hospital as a team-building exercise because you form friendships like no other in that scenario (paintballing would probably be more fun, though). We spend every night staying up late, talking about nothing and everything. We laugh to the point of tears. We swap advice. We celebrate each other's victories, the kind of victories that to most people on the outside wouldn't seem like a big deal (Jackie managed to get out of bed today, three cheers for Jackie everyone), but we know more than most how hard simple tasks can be when you are not feeling well. We order pizza and argue about who is the least socially anxious and therefore the right candidate to go down to get it from the delivery person. We cheer each other up. We don't make a big deal when one of us has a bad day. We sunbathe out in the garden. We watch movies. Plan each other's futures based on what we know of our real lives. A few may or may not sneak out one night and go to Coppers. There is no judgement, no expectation; we can be our true selves when we are together. There is something about living with people who are just as weird as you that really makes you feel at home. Some of these people are still in my life, others I have lost contact with, and unfortunately not all of us made it. The friends I made in that psychiatric hospital are, without doubt, some of the greatest people I have ever met.

Eventually I get tired of living in a mental health unit. The medication has not gotten rid of the voices, my head is foggy and I cannot remember the last time I felt a genuine emotion. I am numb. I am off my head on prescription medication, so I can't feel anything any more. I need to get out of here. I tell Freddie as much and we form a plan. It takes a while for Freddie to stop talking utter nonsense and actually communicate with me enough to help, but once we have learned our lines, I start to act like someone who is getting better.

I talk about my plans for the future: how I am going to walk out of here a new woman, how my treatment has given me a new outlook on life, how from now on I am going to live life to the fullest and embrace this wonderful journey that we call life with a positive mental attitude. I am so happy to be alive –

Freddie: *You're overdoing it. Calm down before they think you're manic.*

'I feel much better. I think I have made enough progress as an inpatient, going home is the next logical step in my recovery. Hopefully, if I continue with my medication and therapy, things will improve further.'

Freddie: *Much better. Gold star.*

They discharge me and I go home.

Chapter 11

Look, I am not going to say the time spent in hospital didn't help. It did, but once again I feel I need to mention how hospitalisation doesn't work as well as the movies make out. I don't walk out of the hospital, say some cheesy line about overcoming my demons and raise my fist in the air in a show of celebration. I get the train home and cry for a week because I miss my hospital friends and I don't know how to function in the real world after becoming institutionalised. I take my medication and beg my doctor to lower the dosage so I can feel human again.

'Are you still hearing voices?'

'Not as much any more.'

'If the voices start to get bad again, we can always go back to the higher dosage. We need to do this slowly and gradually so you don't have another episode of psychosis.'

This is the part I don't understand. All of the mental health professionals, the psychology textbooks and Google searches tell me that my psychosis should come in episodes. I should hear voices and find them distressing, but they should stop with medication and treatment. But I hear them all the time. They never go away. I must be in a psychotic episode permanently, and both doctors and books tell me that someone like me should be in a terrible state given the circumstances. I get depressed, anxious; my mood gets a bit too high; I have suicidal thoughts; I hurt myself to cope, and sometimes I believe silly, impossible things. The voices are all these mental health professionals care about: mentioning them is the only thing that makes them take me seriously. But the voices are the least of my worries. They used to scare me, back when all they did was tell me to kill myself, when they only told me bad things. Still, the other voices, the good ones, are there too. They are a part of me.

When I was in the psychosis programme, they spoke about getting back to what our lives were like 'before' we got sick. I don't have a 'before'; I have always been sick. There were the faceless man and the bad woman, the crows and the pictures, the people and the voices. If I was normal before that, I don't remember it.

I have always had voices in my head. Like the one that sounds like a posh British woman. She has been around since I was small and I adore listening to her Queen's English accent. I can't communicate with her, obviously – only Freddie gets the privilege of conversing with me – but she's cute and I love when she pops up. There is a Scottish man who comes out with some quality one-liners. The majority of my voices sound like people I know or hear on the radio and television. They don't bother me as much as they should and that concerns me.

Am I not schizophrenia-ing, right? Is there even a correct way to be psychotic?

> ## HOW TO BE MENTAL TIP 14
>
> Fuck the textbook versions of your mental illness. Studying psychology does not compare to having a lived experience. You could try to compare a hundred people who have the same illness and I can guarantee you that they would all be different. Don't get hung up like I did over not fitting into the black-and-white terms mental health problems are given.

One thing I learned in hospital is what happens when my mind seems to switch off and a fuzzy cloud surrounds my brain, making my mind feel muddy and slow. It is called 'dissociation', a common side effect of most mental illnesses. When it occurs, your mind drifts away and you stay somewhat present but detached from reality. It's like a fog seeps through your thoughts and you feel like you are dreaming. You are aware of it happening but you cannot pull yourself out of that state. It also ties in with 'depersonalisation', where you feel like you are not connected to yourself, where your body and mind are split into two parts and your limbs may not feel like your own. In this case, it might feel as though your actions don't have consequences because the world around you is not real and any moment now you are going to snap out of it by waking up. Depersonalisation feels as though you are a passenger in your own body. During my time at the hospital, I also learn that there is no such thing as normal, really. 'Neurotypical' is a better word. The term describes people with typical cognitive and developmental disabilities. People who don't have autism, intellectual disabilities or mental illness.

As my medication is reduced, I start to move forward with my life a little bit. I use some of the strategies I learned on my psychosis programme. I can't even remember most of them now, but I know that initially they worked. Then, just as I start to get back on my feet, it all falls apart again.

> **HOW TO BE MENTAL TIP 15**
>
> Sometimes you go to the bad place for reasons that have nothing to do with having a mental illness. Sometimes, life happens and if there is one thing I have learned about life – it isn't fair.

A few months after I get discharged from hospital, Mam's cancer comes back. She has secondary tumours in her lungs despite never having had so much as a single cigarette. At first, we think she has to have chemotherapy, but I am with her when she gets the phone call telling her the cancer isn't as serious as they initially thought and we breathe a sigh of relief. She starts hormone replacement therapy instead. It makes her tired but, overall, she is doing well.

I am at home with her one Wednesday afternoon when she gets a call that Gary has been brought to the doctor's. Apparently, he was hit on the head with something and he needs stitches. We go straight in and the doctor meets us at the door to tell us Gary's skull has been fractured. It turns out that the accident was a lot more serious than we thought. Gary was standing in the school yard when a boy threw a hurley at another lad who caught it and went to throw it back. He missed and it broke on Gary's head instead. There were no teachers around when it happened. Gary's friends helped him inside and the only member of staff they came across was the lady who runs the canteen. She brought him to the doctor's, who realised the seriousness of the situation and called an ambulance.

When we walk in, Gary is lying in the doctor's office with a bandage around his head. He doesn't say much as Mam fusses over him. We ask him what happened but he doesn't answer. He seems stunned, staring into space and looking confused. When the paramedics arrive, they ask Gary for his name.

'It's Luke.'

'Alright Luke,' the paramedic says, 'can you tell us what happened?'

'His name isn't Luke,' Mam says, her face pale. I stand in the corner watching. A voice in my head tells me she wants to go bird watching when she finishes writing her thesis.

'Can you tell me your full name?'

'Luke. Luke Maguire.' Gary seems very sure of this.

The paramedic looks at Mam and she shakes her head. He points at her, 'Do you know who this is?'

'Yeah. It's the man.'

'Can you tell me when your birthday is?'

'Yeah. I can.'

'What is it then?'

'I know when it is.'

'Do you know what date it is?'

Gary gets frustrated. 'Yeah. I know. I know when it is.'

What happens next is like a scene from a horror film.

Gary freezes. He opens his mouth impossibly wide, his jaw making this inhuman-looking movement. His eyes roll back as he convulses on the bed, his limbs contorting, shaking uncontrollably as he froths at the mouth.

Utter mayhem ensues. I am completely useless in these kinds of situations, so I run out of the room and ring Kieran as if he can do something to make everything better. I don't know what is happening and I watch helpless as they load Gary into the ambulance. Before I know it, it has sped off, siren blaring, with Mam and Gary inside. I get a lift to my car and drive up to Cork University Hospital on autopilot. I pray to a god I don't even believe in not to take another brother from me. This morning, everything was normal. How did things go from zero to hundred so quickly?

Freddie: *Because Gary's head cracked open.*

'Stop it.'

Freddie: *Like an egg. Humpty Dumpty sat on the wall, he had a great fall. His brains went splat across the pavement. Do you think Gary is going to be brain dead?*

'Shut up, shut up, shut up. Why are you being so mean?'

Freddie: *Because I can.*

The next few hours are terrifying. Dad and Jamie come

to the hospital. They show us his scans. He has a compound depressed fracture of the left frontal region with intracranial air and contusions. In plain English, he fractured his skull and the part that broke pierced through the spongy part that sits in between the skull and the brain. He has to go for emergency surgery. I see his injury when they unwrap the bandages, it looks like he has a hole in his head.

After he wakes up from surgery, he seems to be doing reasonably well at first. The poor boy who threw the hurley comes to see him. I feel sorry for him; it was a freak accident and he wasn't to know what would happen. I can only imagine the guilt he is feeling. Gary is never the same after the accident. He has an acquired brain injury, which impacts every aspect of his life from now on. He has seizures and headaches. Some of these seizures take place in very public places like school or when he's out with friends. I find myself driving after an ambulance again one day after a particularly bad one. He played a lot of sports before the accident but that all has to stop.

He develops post-traumatic stress disorder (PTSD) and ends up spending a few months in the adolescent version of the same psychiatric hospital I was in. PTSD is a mental health condition triggered by a terrifying event – either experiencing or witnessing it. Symptoms can include uncontrollable thoughts about the event, poor memory, startle reflex, intrusive memories, flashbacks, apathy and nightmares. Gary can go from being fine to a state of distress and hyper-vigilance, usually triggered by hearing an ambulance siren in real life or on the television. He is impossible to calm down when he gets in these states. The part of the brain that was injured, the frontal lobe, is responsible for controlling our personalities, our emotions, memory, judgement, skills such as problem-solving and our ability to communicate. Damage to the frontal lobe can cause a range of issues, but mainly an inability to understand social cues, impaired moral judgement, aggression, impulsivity and loss of empathetic reasoning. Gary's brain injury comes with an entirely new personality. He is cold, uncaring, angry, violent and cannot comprehend the difference between right and wrong. He makes poor decisions and lashes out at everyone around him. He goes through hell and so do we.

A year later, my grandmother Phyllis, who has had Alzheimer's disease for eight years, passes away. It's a slow process. She forgets who we are, she forgets who she is and eventually she forgets how to swallow food or water; there is nothing that can be done to keep her alive then. At least she is too far gone to know what's going on – it's not a nice way to go. The doctor says he wishes there were an injection he could give her to speed things up. The human body can survive a surprisingly long time without any food. One day Mam and I take a break from our bedside vigil and go for a walk. 'If I ever get to the stage where I have no quality of life, do me a favour and shoot me,' she says. 'I never want you to have to look after me, it's one of my biggest fears, having my children care for me like that.' Phyllis slips away a few weeks later, finally at peace.

At this stage I have moved out of home, and I work on a make-up counter at a department store. When I was a child, I was always the slow one, the one left behind, or, as Mam's friend once put it, I never 'thrived'. But the beauty of being an adult is that I am in the same league as everyone else; no one has any idea what they are doing. I remember crying at Mam in hospital one time that I was never going to be able to live in the real world, as I knew nothing about taxes or mortgages. How would I ever be able to pay bills or learn any of the critical life skills that are required when you become a certain age? When I leave the nest and gain a bit of independence, however, I discover that everyone is just as lost and confused as I am. We are all just making it up as we go along.

Adulthood is a lot harder than we make it out to be. We would be much better off if we were honest and said, 'I don't know what I'm doing either', to each other more. I still ring Mam five times a day because I am as needy as ever, but it feels good to live a life that is more than what was expected of me in the past. When I was diagnosed I thought: *that's it, all downhill from here, I will only get more unwell and more dependent.* I am by no means completely better, not even close, but I'm learning how to live with my illness. Still, my early twenties are full of relapses.

HOW TO BE MENTAL TIP 16

Recovery is not linear. You get better just to get sick again and then you get better again. Around and around that cycle you shall go. It's okay, it happens to us all; the trick is to learn from relapse and establish what you can do to improve things before they get really bad.

Chapter 12

It is Christmas 2013 when Mam gets unexpectedly rushed to hospital. She has tumours in her brain. I know what this means, she knows, everyone knows – but we don't acknowledge it. Everything changes after that. I always hear people talking about cancer in those campaigns like it is a person. Stand up to cancer, tell cancer who is boss, kick cancer's ass. I feel like cancer is a person too, and, oddly enough, it now feels like a family member. The day the disease spreads to her brain, it is as if cancer has walked into our kitchen, put its feet upon our table and demanded to be part of the family. It weaves its way through our home and poisons everything it touches. The black sheep of the family, the toxic member everyone shuns but has to put up with. Every time we sit around the table for a meal, every event, every conversation, every time we exchange presents on Christmas morning, every time someone blows out their birthday candles, it is there, demanding our attention.

We are sitting eating dinner, talking loudly in an attempt to drown out the sounds of Mam getting sick in the kitchen sink. I walk into her bedroom to find her having a seizure on the bed. Her hair falls out and she puts on her wig and acts as though nothing is wrong. We are never permitted to talk about what might happen, she won't hear of it. Apart from when she goes through a phase of hating me. She looks at me like she detests me; nothing I do for her is right. I know, in hindsight, that when someone is sick, they often take it out on the people closest to them, but in the moment it hurts when she says I don't do enough for her.

My commute to work takes two hours with morning traffic and it is an hour and a half back in the evenings. When I am on a late followed by an early, I get home in time for a nap before getting up to go back again. I get a text from one of Mam's friends one day asking me where I am and why I'm not with my mother. 'I'm in work,' I text back, 'like everyone else in my family, I have to go to work so I can pay my rent.'

That's the thing. Mam has cancer for years, it is not like on TV when everyone drops everything and gathers around her bedside. Life has to go on to some degree. I remember someone in work saying to me how she can't understand how I still come in every day. If it was her mother, she would take compassionate leave. I try to explain the situation – taking years of compassionate leave isn't exactly practical. I do end up asking for a few days. After my request I get summoned to the office by a manager and she asks me how long my mother's condition could go on for and whether there will be an end point.

'Are you asking me when she is going to die?'

She says that is not how she would like to put it, but yes essentially, she wants to know: have the doctors given my mother weeks or months? She has a business to run, and the more time I take off, the more money the counter loses.

In all the time Mam has been sick I have never spoken to or seen a doctor, let alone some sort of team that keeps us informed every step of the way. So I have no idea how long my mother has left, but when the time comes, I hopefully will be able to give enough notice so I can attend the funeral and get back to what is really important. Peddling over-priced cosmetics.

I am only back on the floor half an hour when I am summoned yet again, this time by a more senior manager, who apologises. Apparently, he had asked the other manager to check up on me out of concern and she misinterpreted what he meant.

Mam tells me about how amazing everyone else is. One of her friends called to the house with a box of chocolates, another friend made her a blanket, one took her for lunch. Jamie lives in the same city where I work and he comes down to see her once during the week and again on the weekends. Nothing I do is enough. I finish work and collect Gary from town. I try to spend as much time with him and Mam as I can. I go home and see Kieran briefly before going to bed to stare at the four walls until it is time to get up. I am completely exhausted and emotionally drained.

One night, I sit on the floor and look up to the ceiling. 'Please,' I say aloud to some unknown being, 'can you give me a break? Just stop making bad stuff happen. I can't take any more.' Not even a minute later my phone buzzes with a Facebook message from someone I don't know. 'Check on your brother. He's taken an overdose.'

This happens a lot. Gary has not been doing well mentally and it is not uncommon for me to get a text from one of his friends, telling me to make sure he pukes up whatever pills he has taken.

The breaking point comes when I stay at my parents' home for a night because I have to bring Gary for an appointment in the morning. At 4 a.m. I go downstairs to check on Mam and I hear her banging around in the kitchen in the morning. There's a mess left over from dinner and this is somehow my fault. I arrived just before midnight and went straight to bed, so the mess couldn't possibly be mine, but this information is irrelevant to her.

'Why are you angry at me all the time? Why is everything my fault?'

'Because I have cancer and you're not doing enough to help me,' she says.

We really get into it then. There are tears from us both. I reach boiling point and say the worst thing I have ever said to anyone, ever. She talks about how good her friends are, how they visit and check up on her. 'It's easy for them to come out once a week with chocolates and a smile and then they can fuck off back to their own lives and their own families. They're not stuck with you all the time like I am.'

My words hang in the air for a long silent pause. I try to

take them back but it's too late. I didn't mean for it to come out so brutally. Her friends have been so supportive, but none of them are her daughter; they can go home to their own families whenever they want, but for us – my dad, Jamie, Gary and me – it is constant.

We sit in the kitchen until the sun comes up. I apologise for being so harsh. Mam explains how she is frustrated with not being able to do things herself, and how the frustration turns to anger, which she doesn't mean to direct at me. I am in no place to judge, considering I spent most of my teenage years screaming at her for daring to care about my well-being. We promise to go easier on one another. We hug it out and put that unpleasant time behind us.

Gary gets worse, as does Mam's health. It becomes our normal, though, just like my schizophrenia, which, if you were wondering, is as prominent as ever. But the bad voices are now totally gone, completely replaced by much nicer voices. There is a woman with a strong Newcastle accent who speaks more than Freddie does, although never directly to me. She just narrates what is going on in my world and gives her opinion on proceedings. The delusions are still there, though; they try to creep in and mess with my common sense. I still get the feeling of being watched all the time, that never goes away. I still check my food for poison and my room for recording devices, but it's not the same as before.

I have become better at distinguishing between what is genuinely real and what is my illness playing tricks on me. I have found a balance between the two worlds, the real one and the psychosis one. The voices do not bother me as much, their non-intrusive nature now is easy to live with compared to what I was dealing with before. I always say I am lucky in a sense. As I developed my illness at such a young age, I have had longer to learn how to live with it. I cannot imagine how hard it must be to go from being neurotypical and living a normal life to being plunged into a world with voices and paranoia with no warning. I don't miss having a normal mind because I never had one. Don't get me wrong, it isn't easy by any means, but I know deep down that my dreams of outgrowing it are unlikely to happen and so this sort of balance is the best I can hope for.

HOW TO BE MENTAL TIP 17

Acceptance is *everything*. Having a psychotic disorder has impacted every single part of my life in some way or another. Everyone who is diagnosed with any kind of long-term mental health problem goes through a sort of grieving process for what might have been. Glorifying how life would have looked if we never got sick. Don't get me wrong, I'm sure it would be much easier and better, but it is what it is. I could spend every day feeling sorry for myself but life will pass me by and I will have achieved nothing.

If Mam's attitude towards cancer has taught me anything, it is that no matter what happens to you, it is how you deal with it that is important. She walks out of every appointment with bad news. She says, 'I want to be better, there are so many things I want to do, I want to be healthy but I'm not. That's not where I am right now but I will get there. I'm not going to waste my time feeling sorry for myself any more, I have to live in the now.'

She does this exercise, which I still do to this day. The same one she tried to teach me before I went to hospital and got diagnosed. Every day you set yourself a certain amount of time – ten minutes to an hour – whatever suits you. It is your allocated time to be negative, to feel sorry for yourself, to be angry. You can think about all the horrible things you want but, as soon as your time is up, you have to move on and think positive thoughts. It takes practice, but as soon as you start thinking negatively remind yourself that this kind of thinking isn't allowed outside of your allocated time, and that time will come around tomorrow when you can think as negatively as you want. I'm making it sound easy, like one of those people who hear you have mental health problems and ask you if you've tried just not being depressed, as if it's that simple. I know it's hard to think positively when you are in the bad place, but you can try that exercise, even if only for a week. If it doesn't work then, fair enough, it's not for you, but there is no harm in trying.

Chapter 13

Australia keeps coming up as a topic of conversation. Kieran doesn't want to go. I want to but am afraid of leaving Mam and Gary given the way they are. Mam is desperate for me to go. She has this positive outlook that she is going to get better, though I don't see how that is possible – not that I ever say this to her.

There is something else at the forefront of my mind right now. Ever since I was diagnosed with schizophrenia, I have become more aware of the stigma that surrounds it. Mental illness in general is stigmatised, but psychotic disorders seem to get it the worst. Every mental health awareness campaign seems to centre around depression and anxiety; I don't see any other illnesses mentioned as much. I see people sharing 'It's okay not to be okay' posts on Facebook, including some people who laughed at me for having psychosis. When I hear people discuss mental health it seems they have the impression that any of the less-common illnesses are what the real crazy people have.

I can see where that idea comes from. After all, the media only seem to talk about schizophrenia when it is in relation to a crime. It is important to cover facts; a person committing a violent crime is, of course, news. Mention that the person in question has schizophrenia by all means. A crime has happened, there are victims here and their family, as well as the public, need to be informed of the incident and to be told how it can be prevented from happening again. My problem is the way in which a lot of these stories are covered. It is made to seem as though schizophrenia can make anyone who has it violent. If someone is violent and evil by nature, schizophrenia is not going to help matters, of course, but the majority of us have never had a violent thought towards others in our lives. We are statistically more likely to be victims of a crime and we are more likely to have suicidal rather than homicidal thoughts. Whenever a person goes on a shooting spree and this is blamed on mental illness, the idea that 'mentally ill monsters' exist is encouraged, or, as Donald Trump put it: 'mental illness pulls the trigger not the gun'. Some people do not want to believe that true evil exists in the world. When someone commits an act of terrorism, a shooting, a massacre, mental illness or their religious beliefs are not the cause or reason. These are individuals with a hatred inside of them, which they express through violence.

Movies and television shows are the worst offenders. Even more liberties are taken when it comes to fiction. The majority of such movies seem to be horribly misinformed. Sometimes it seems as if no research has been done whatsoever. Characters with schizophrenia either seem to be violent or geniuses. Lifetimes are spent in mental hospitals. Medication cures all and if you stop taking your pills a bout of violent crime is inevitable. Another classic is using the it-was-him-the-whole-time 'plot twist' – we see that one time and time again. The character realising at the end of the movie that it was them who had been getting up to all sorts of wacky adventures and that they have a split personality, which is often wrongly referred to as schizophrenia. The entertainment industry and media can be misleading and this results in the general population becoming more misinformed about what psychosis actually is.

Schizophrenia has become an excuse for inexcusable actions and is constantly used as a scapegoat. It is a lot harder to tell someone and get help for a condition when it carries the weight of such strong misconceptions. Every time schizophrenia is used for sensationalism it sets us back. Not every person with schizophrenia spends their life in a mental hospital. Medication is not some required-by-law absolute must. An awful lot of us go on to lead normal, successful lives. Schizophrenia may be an incurable disease, but that does not mean it is unmanageable. Stigma has delayed my recovery many times. I am usually okay with having a psychotic illness, but sometimes other people's ignorance can change that. When I hear someone describe schizophrenia as multiple-personality disorder, or use the word schizo, or misuse the word psychotic, it takes away a little bit of the resilience and self-acceptance I have worked so hard to build up. Every time I see my mental health problem used in the media as an excuse or explanation for a person's crime or wrongdoing, it can bring on feelings of shame and a need to justify my illness to those who tar us all with the same brush. I wish someone would speak out and talk about schizophrenia. I want people to understand what it actually is and I want more awareness around it. Then it hits me, an impossible thought that I brush off until I can't any more. If I want the attitude towards schizophrenia to change, there is no use sitting back and waiting for someone else to do it. At the same time, it sounds ridiculous, who would even care about my story?

Freddie: *Oh, just get fucking on with it, will you?*

I have zero expectations when I write a little piece on my experience. I keep it short, cover the main events: how young I was when it started, all the way up to my most recent hospital stay and how I am doing now. I look over it and send it into Her.ie before really giving myself a chance to think about it. I probably should have taken longer; I literally had it written and sent in the space of an hour. I blame Freddie's constant nagging for that. I get an email back early the next morning, asking for my full name and a photograph. I ring Mam in a panic – she always wanted me to keep it private – but the second I tell her what I have done, she tells me to go for it. She explains to me later that since her cancer became what it is now, she knows the importance of raising awareness.

I know there is a chance it could ruin my life; I might struggle with employment or people might look at me differently, but, then, I have always been looked at as someone who is different. At least now I can be open about the reason why.

Looking back, it was the best decision I ever made. I never could have predicted how much one choice would change my life. I don't know where I would be now if I hadn't taken that leap into the unknown.

HOW TO BE MENTAL TIP 18

Life happens outside of your comfort zone. There is a lot to be said for 'feeling the fear and doing it anyway'.

The article goes up on 19 February 2014. Twenty-four hours later, I sit staring at my phone as the notifications and messages continue to stream in. I can hardly believe the support, the kind comments, the positive messages. My inbox is flooded with people who have psychosis, bipolar disorder, BPD, depression, OCD or anxiety. The diagnosis doesn't matter, they all want the same thing – to be understood.

The question that I get the most, and the one that breaks my heart every time, is 'How do I make my family or friends understand my mental health problems? How can I show them that I don't want to be this way? How can I make them see I can't snap out of it?' I never know the answer. All I have is:

HOW TO BE MENTAL TIP 19

Some people are lost causes. You can spend your life trying to make them understand but they never will, unless they go through it themselves. It is not your responsibility to take the weight of their ignorance.

The people I speak to are mothers, fathers, teachers, doctors, solicitors, shop assistants, hurlers, hairdressers, chefs, plumb-

ers, researchers, radio DJs, students, carpenters, factory workers, footballers, make-up artists, dentists – there is no specific
background, gender, sexual orientation or race. Mental illness
does not discriminate, it can go after any of us. There is only
one particular pattern among the people who reach out to me.
Most of them are men. Men who are too afraid of being seen
as less of a man if they ask for help. Men who think going to
counselling is a sign of weakness. Men who are terrified of
being 'found out'. I hear from people all over the world, but
I often speak to men who live in my town, whom I went to
school with but never really talked to, men who spend their
Friday nights drinking pints with the lads and their Sundays
out on the field with a hurley or a football, men who have always been seen as confident and happy but who message me
in the dead of night to tell me how they can cry every day for
weeks and don't know why. They don't want to be seen going in
or out of a local therapist's office, they don't want to be laughed
at or told to man up. It makes me sad to see people waste years
of their life not getting the help they need. No one goes to the
funeral of someone who dies by suicide and says, 'Wasn't he
a great lad? Not telling anyone what was going on. He didn't
talk about his feelings, let himself suffer, all the way up to the
very end, fair play to him.'

There is hope in a lot of the stories. I get messages from
those who have turned it all around and come out the other
side. They still feel it – once you experience mental ill health
it never truly goes away – but they have learned how to be
happy, even if their minds are a little broken sometimes.

I never thought sharing my story would lead to so many conversations with people who are just like me. Speaking to them helps me to tell myself the same things I tell them. Your illness is not your fault. It is okay to have bad days. You have done a wonderful job of surviving despite all the obstacles thrown at you.

I do my first of many radio interviews shortly afterwards. It feels like it's happening to someone else. I go with the flow, doing more interviews, writing more articles, while I watch from a distance impostor-syndrome style and think, *is this real life?*

I get media trained. I say yes to everything at the start. I do all the big shows. I find myself at RTÉ, Today FM, Newstalk. I am asked to give a talk at a charity event. I have never given any kind of talk before, unless you want to count the public speaking exam in speech and drama where ten-year-old me clutched her notes and in a shaky voice told a couple of bored-looking examiners everything that my dial-up internet research had told me about earthquakes. I say yes before I can think about it much, which has pretty much been my strategy so far. I stand in a room full of people and tell them my story. I answer questions at the end. It is straightforward enough so I do it again. And again. And again. I don't get nervous, which is strange, not even a little bit. Freddie doesn't let me.

Freddie: *Fuck it. Just go for it. What's the worst that could happen? It's an hour of your life and then it's done. You've gotten through worse. This is the easy bit.*

He is right. How scary can a live interview be when I once

lay in bed and watched the room fill with people who stood staring at me until I put the covers over my head? If I can listen to a voice telling me to kill myself, surely I can answer a few questions with Ryan Tubridy. This becomes my way of thinking and Freddie is all for it.

Talk about my personal problems on a stage in front of a hundred people?

'Not a bother.'

Freddie: *Piece of piss.*

Someone dropped out of an interview and we need you to go live in ten minutes.

'Grand. Put me through there and I'll get it done before my lunch break is over.'

Freddie: *That's what I like to hear.*

Would you be interested in doing a bit of guest lecturing for my psychology students?

'No problem at all.'

Freddie: *That FETAC Level 5 may not be a PhD, but it counts for something.*

'I don't even recognise myself any more, Freddie. I never thought I would be capable of any of this.'

Freddie: *Not gonna lie, neither did I. I only told you to go for it because I thought you'd fuck it all up and I would have some light entertainment. But go you. Have the goldest of stars.*

It never affects me when it comes to employment. My manager calls me up to his office and says he was surprised to hear my voice on 98FM this morning. I did that interview pulled in on a lay-by on my way to work.

Freddie: *Oh, you're in trouble now.*

'Yeah that was me,' I say.

He informs me that he was surprised again to find my face looking back at him when he opened the *Independent*, along with my accompanying article. He ends up being nice about it, if annoyed that I didn't tell him I had schizophrenia so they could be aware of it. He seems to find it funny how there were no signs. This is how it is with some people; with others I get 'I always knew there was something wrong with you'. When I change to a different store, my new manager reacts to the news of me having schizophrenia the same way you would expect if I had told her I have asthma.

I am contacted by an organisation called See Change, which aims to reduce the stigma around mental health. They run the Green Ribbon campaign every May, which raises awareness and encourages people to be more open. They ask me to be a part of their ambassador programme, which is a group of people with lived experience sharing their stories. I meet many amazing and inspirational people through this. Rita and Kelley, who live close to me, organise many events that raise awareness. Rick, who had been diagnosed with bipolar and borderline-personality disorder after many suicide attempts, including jumping off a building, which broke his back and legs, has now dedicated his life to the cause. He is one of the greatest advocates I know.

Then there is Derek Devoy, who set up a suicide prevention initiative called Taxi Watch, where taxi drivers complete a course with the HSE designed to help them spot people who are in distress and know how to talk to someone who is suicidal. Derek has been through depression himself. Years ago, he would get ready to go to work in the morning but retreat back to bed as soon as his wife left with the children, which left her unaware of how bad things were getting. Eventually the pretence of going to work was exposed when he fell into debt and was threatened with repossession of his house. After a back injury, caused by a crash with a drunk driver, he fell deeper into depression and made the decision to end his life. After a few attempts, Derek got the help he needed and his condition improved. One night, while driving his taxi around Kilkenny, he saw a man getting ready to jump from a bridge. When Derek stopped to talk to the man, he told him the bank was repossessing his house. After Derek contacted the emergency services, the man was seen to, and an hour later Derek encountered another man about to jump from the same spot. A group of lads drove past in a car and shouted, 'Do a flip'. Derek started Taxi Watch then. His suicide prevention project has spread across the country and the scheme has directly intervened in over 200 suicide attempts.

A woman pulls me aside after a talk one day and says, 'You better not get sick again; it won't send a good message to the rest of us then.'

I know, instantly, that this is going to become a problem later. It can get really overwhelming when strangers are looking for help and I try to explain how I'm not equipped to do much for them. I think some people forget I'm mentally ill too, and they can get annoyed when I don't get back to them quickly enough. They don't understand that I am going through my own issues sometimes.

Some of the questions people ask are inappropriate, especially on nights out when their inhibitions are lowered. 'Are you even allowed to have children?' I get this on more than one occasion, along with 'I thought schizophrenics had to take their medication?' I have to explain that there is no such thing as a schizophrenia police ready to whisk me away for not taking meds or for possibly making a little human one day. To be fair, though, I had thought this about myself when I was first diagnosed.

HOW TO BE MENTAL TIP 20

Not all ignorance is malicious. I prefer people to ask questions and have a genuine curiosity. If I don't tell them, I cannot expect them to know. Just because a question may not be worded right doesn't mean it isn't valid. Answering every question, even the wildly inappropriate ones, helps to reduce the stigma.

The funny thing is, every interviewer wants the success story, how I am fully recovered and living a psychosis-free life. I have to explain that I am still psychotic, just dealing with it better. I don't mention Freddie. It is one thing hearing voices, but giving them names seems like another level of crazy. I am open about my illness, but since going public I have learned that it is a bit like when you start a new relationship: you have to keep some of the crazy inside and let it out in bits and pieces, not all at once.

Whenever I am asked if any of my voices have a name, the answer I give is always no.

Freddie: *Well fuck you too.*

Chapter 14

It's June 2015 and the day we leave for Australia has finally arrived. I sit on my mother's bed and ask her a question that she must have heard a thousand times by now. 'Yes, Nicola, I promise you if anything happens, we will tell you.'

Kieran and I moved back to our respective homes eight months ago to save and spend time with our families before we left. 'You need to live your own life. All I want is for you to be happy. This is everything you want; I need to see you do what you were always meant to do.'

I have agonised over leaving her, leaving Gary. I have three fears.

1) I'll hate Australia and my lifelong dream wasn't for me after all

2) Mam will get sicker and

3) Gary will become worse.

On the drive to the airport, I ask my dad the same question. 'I keep telling you, Nic, if anything happens or if you need to come home, I will tell you. I'll keep you informed every step of the way.'

Leaving is the biggest relief of my life. No more sickness, no more looking after Gary. I had an incident in work recently where I was wrongly accused of doing something. The formal apology I received after the investigation was nice but the damage was done and I couldn't bear to work with the person who lied about me to get herself out of trouble. Then there is the person who I don't name, who, seven years later, is still telling anyone who will listen how my mental illness is all for attention. I have lost more friends than I can count to this person. None of that matters now. It is all gone. Gone. Gone. Gone. Far away.

The more distance I put between myself and home, the freer I feel. I was always told running away from your problems is a bad thing until a therapist told me that I can't expect to recover from trauma when I am still surrounded by it; you have to take yourself away from what hurts you in order to heal. And heal I do. As soon as we land, I feel as though I am exactly where I am supposed to be, which is an entirely new feeling.

Later on, my dad will tell me how they waited for what they thought was the inevitable hysterical phone call that we messed up somewhere and we were homeless and jobless on the streets of Sydney, but it never comes. We stay with Clíona, who used to babysit me as a child, for the first week. She shows us around, gets us set up with bank accounts and all the other important stuff. We find an apartment and get jobs.

And I mean jobs – I get several offers in the first few weeks and have to pick one. It turns out that beauty therapists who specialise in eyebrows are in high demand here. I turn down an offer every other week and I wonder what kind of land of wonderment this is where you don't even have to look for a job, it finds you.

Making friends in Sydney is a lot easier than in Ireland because expats tend to stick together. June is the middle of winter in Australia, of course, but it's still warm. We live in a studio apartment that has been infested with cockroaches for so long that everyone in the building accepts them as part of the furniture. Bondi Beach is a quick walk down the road and the bus stop is right outside our door so we can't complain. We go into a bubble, the Aussie bubble we call it. Our little safe haven where the problems from home no longer dominate our every waking thought. I am happier than I have ever been. Then there is Kieran, who has developed mental health problems of his own in recent years. Anxiety and OCD to be specific. We once had a panic attack at the same time – maybe I am contagious or something. But neither of us have had any since we got here.

We got engaged two years ago. It is lovely knowing someone is happy to spend the rest of their life with me. We have been together a long time now and taking the next step was inevitable. The shit thing about getting engaged, though, was how some people praised Kieran for wanting to be with someone like me. 'You are so lucky he stuck by you, most men would run a mile', 'Aren't you so good to stay with that poor sick girl?' 'It must be hard to live with, fair play to you for seeing past her condition.' This does not go down well with me.

No one at the time knew about Kieran's problems, about how it works both ways. They assume our relationship is some sort of carer-and-patient situation. One of the most stigmatising things about having any kind of disability is people pitying you or thinking there is nothing more about you beyond your condition. As if it would be impossible for Kieran to love me for me – my diagnosis must get in the way somehow. After our engagement no one was more annoyed about this than Mam, who went out of her way on several occasions to remind people that Kieran is very lucky to have me too.

Since we have been in Australia she seems to be doing well. She sends me texts with positive affirmations every day and we talk on the phone regularly. She tells me Gary is doing fine and her treatment is going well. Kieran and I were supposed to get married that summer but we'd cancelled it, as I wanted to wait until Mam was in a better place and we had already prioritised the cost of moving to Australia over a wedding – we weren't able to afford both.

Mam gets in touch on the date that was supposed to be our wedding. She says it's okay to feel sad about it but what I'm doing is far more important than a day out and a piece of paper. She tells me she is in hospital but it's not serious. 'There is a bit of nerve damage in my foot, I'll have to stay here until it heals but it won't be for long, I have a wheelchair to get around but other than that I have no news.' The only person from home I seem to hear from is Mam. Most of my messages to the rest of them go ignored.

Freddie doesn't acknowledge Australia. I don't know why but he never mentions how we live in a different country now. He has carried on, business as usual, since we arrived. I gave up on trying to work out how Freddie operates a long time ago.

I am lying in bed one night, trying to get to sleep. Freddie is talking about something stupid as he always does. There are a few other voices: the posh woman is there, a man and a woman who sound like Americans are having a conversation about directions to somewhere. There are street noises. The Americans are talking about a doctor. A truck whizzes through my mind. I can hear what sounds like a large body of water, maybe a waterfall, but from far away. And then with no warning at all, as if someone flicked a switch or pulled a plug, they stop. All of them, including Freddie, the voices, the noises, they stop dead. I wait for them to come back. Seconds go by and then I hear something else. It's new. It is an empty dead sound. Silence. This is what silence sounds like.

I shake Kieran awake. Still half-asleep, but alarmed, he asks what is wrong. He probably thinks I am being attacked by one of the cockroaches again.

'I can't hear anything.'

He studies me with one eye open for a moment. I know I am wide eyed and borderline hysterical, waiting for him to understand the gravity of the situation.

'I should hope not at this hour.' He tries to go back to sleep.

'No, no, no. You don't understand. I can't hear anything.' I tap my head.

He's fully awake then. 'Fuck off?'

'I know, they were all there and then they just … stopped. Like a switch going off. I can't hear anything at all.'

I'm excited at first, I get Kieran to keep talking and his voice sounds different without all the background noise I'm used to. My own voice sounds different or maybe I'm imagining it. I abandon a desire to go outside to see what it sounds like out there because I don't think any resident of Bondi out late is going to be comfortable with seeing a woman in her pyjamas out on the street muttering to herself that the voices have finally gone. I put music on but there isn't much of a difference in how it sounds. The only music I have on my phone is that album U2 gave everyone for free so maybe it is because I am not familiar with the song.

The novelty starts to wear off then. I don't like it, I decide; silence has a cold, hollow sound.

'Fucking hell. Is this what you've all been hearing all along?' I ask Kieran. 'You poor thing, this is horrible.'

It lasts for seventeen minutes. They don't come back as suddenly as they left. They slowly trickle in, one by one, until the whole team is back.

'Where did you go?'

Freddie: *Nowhere. Where did you go?*

'The same, I suppose.'

Freddie: *Don't do that again.*

***

It's funny how I spent such a large part of my life believing that there was such a thing as normal people who didn't have problems. A younger, self-absorbed version of me thought I had the worst problems in the world. Everyone has imperfect parts in their life; we're all fighting some sort of battle. Whether our problems are big or small, we all have our demons. But I thought I had come out the other side, living my Australian dream, doing what I had always wanted to do, on the route to happiness.

I look at my life now as broken into two parts – before and after. I had no idea on a normal Sunday watching TV on the couch in our apartment in Sydney, blissfully living in the 'before', that I was about to be swiftly catapulted into the 'after'.

I am on the phone to someone back home. We're catching up on trivial stuff. Kieran sits beside me, playing a game on his phone. The lads from down the road are on the TV, saving someone's life on Bondi Rescue. Freddie is asking me if we are doing anything later. I ask about my mam.

'Look, I can imagine it's hard for you over there not being able to do anything. It's just hard for us all having to deal with the shit here.'

They are rambling on and I am clueless to what they are talking about.

'Is everything okay? Is my mam alright?'

'As good as she can be, I suppose. It's tough going, though.'

I make eye contact with Kieran and give him a pointed look. 'What?' he mouths, going back to his phone when I don't respond.

'I mean, I don't know if anyone has said anything to you about coming home but I wouldn't leave it too late.'

The blood drains from my body. I hear words like 'goodbye' 'time' and 'not long'. A voice in my head is talking about how a haircut can change the shape of someone's face.

'Your brother decided not to bring his wedding forward. No point in rushing things, it was a nice idea but sure she wouldn't even be able to enjoy the day. It's sad that she won't ever see her son get married but what can you do.'

Freddie: *You can do this; you've had plenty of practice. Just continue on as normal. Keep your voice light. That's it. Start wrapping it up. Say you have to go and you'll talk to them soon. Hang up. Hang up. Hang up.*

I follow his instructions on autopilot.

Freddie: *Breezy does it, nothing's wrong, everything is fine. You're doing great. Right talk to you soon. Say the twenty-two byes you Irish like to say before you hang up. And done. Gold star.*

I stare through the television. There is an insurance ad on. Time stands still. Kieran is still sitting there, oblivious to my world shattering beside him. A cockroach scurries across the floor and our Brazilian neighbours are shouting at each other in the alleyway. It is evening time and still bright out. The phone remains in my hand, I've not dropped it in slow motion the way they do in films. The words swim around me. 'Won't ever see her son get married but what can you do.' She's dying. Dying. Fucking dying. Not sick or having a funny turn or whatever lies I have been fed for however long, she is going to die.

Kieran asks if everything is okay at home. I tell him my mam is going to die. Saying the words out loud for the first time feels strange. He thinks I misunderstood what the person meant, there has to be a reasonable explanation. I make the phone calls. I ring Sylvia, I ring my dad. It is a long time before I get the full story. Two weeks after we landed in Sydney, the cancer spread to her nervous system. There was nothing anyone could do after that. She has not been in hospital; she is in a hospice. She doesn't have a sore foot, she is paralysed from the chest down, she is slowly going blind, she is not going to get better, she is going to die. She insisted that no one tell me and everyone has gone along with it. Her birthday party that they threw her a few weeks ago was a farewell party. All her friends and all our family gathered around, making her final wishes come true, and I was here. On the other side of the world, unaware that my mother's final months were happening without me.

Her way of dealing with things is to pretend she is going to be fine. This is why my dad is telling me I can't come home, because my sudden return might scare her into reality. I don't care, I need to see her, I have to say goodbye. Kieran is in as much shock as I am. This can't be happening. How could they have gone all this time without telling us? There were signs, I think now, looking back, the way phone calls and texts had been ignored. Everyone must have been avoiding me like the plague in case they inadvertently told me, like that person had done. The only person who has been consistently answering the phone to me is Mam and that's because, in her mind, there isn't anything to tell me. She still believes everything is going to be okay, that she has a future.

After a sleepless night we take the next day off work. I have my dad half-convinced that I need to make a visit home. The plan is to go by myself, see her, spend some time at her side and fly back to Australia until there is more news. I can't fly to Ireland for a few more weeks. Life is never that simple, there are arrangements to be made.

Flying home all of a sudden will definitely scare her but if she is given some warning about my 'holiday' she can expect me and get excited about it without suspecting anything being amiss. At least that is what my dad tells me is the best course of action. I share the news with some of our friends but it still doesn't seem real, like I'm talking about somebody else's mother. It all seems so far away, probably because it is. Mam's time is ticking away and I feel like I might as well be on another planet.

There is a lunar eclipse that night. We head down to the beach to see it. We sit in our usual spot on the grassy hill. Mam's love for the sea view at home has always seemed a bit silly to me but now I understand why a view can mean so much. When we sit here, we can see the beach, the sea, the cliffs, and it has become my favourite place. We sit and look at the moon, blood-red in the sky. It is the most beautiful sight I have ever seen.

Kieran puts his arm around me, pulling me close to him. A tear escapes down my cheek. I might be pretending to myself that I am only going home for a visit, but I know deep down our time here is over.

Chapter 15

Nothing could have prepared me for what she looks like now. I don't know who the person in the bed is, but she is not my mother. She is not the woman I waved goodbye to just a few months ago. She looks different, far worse than I have ever seen her, but it is not just this that shocks me. My mam is like a child, or someone heading into the worst stages of Alzheimer's disease. The drugs don't help in this regard – she swigs from a bottle of morphine, there doesn't seem to be a limit to how much she can have. It takes me longer than I care to admit to work out that the reason she has an endless supply of hardcore pain relief is that it doesn't matter if she takes dangerous amounts, as she will be dead soon anyway.

Her voice is barely a whisper, as she struggles to string a sentence together, giving me an answer as to why she has ignored most of my calls. I am under strict instructions to pretend this is a casual visit home. I am struggling to see what the issue is, as if I told her that I'd discovered how to teleport and beamed myself home she would probably believe me, she is that far gone.

I have left Kieran back in Sydney. It is going to be the longest we have ever been apart: twelve days. I ring him when I am outside the hospice. It is morning in Australia and I can hear the sounds of the city in the background as he makes his way to work.

'Worse than you thought?' he asks.

I tell him how bad it is. Everything is bad here. It only takes a minute of being in Gary's presence to know that things have gotten a lot worse there too. Another secret kept from me. As the days go on, and I start to run out of time, I know what I have to do. I think I have always known. From that horrible moment when I connected the dots and realised that my mother was dying, I knew that we would have to come home for good, that Australia was over. The bubble has burst.

I spent my whole life working towards it: the image of finally leaving and getting my chance to go to the other side of the world and start a new life had gotten me through the worst of times. It didn't matter how many breakdowns I had, how much I hurt, how often I reached my lowest lows, the dream of moving to Australia had motivated me, kept me going, given me a reason not to give up. It was my chance to do what I wanted to do for once, my chance to be happy. I got five months.

Telling Kieran is not easy. He never wanted to go in the first place. I dragged him all the way over there, he gave it his best shot and is happy with the life we have been making for ourselves. Now I have to go and ruin it. He understands, of course he does; he is ready to uproot his life for me again.

Explaining to Mam that I will probably be back soon is not as easy. I come out with a big elaborate story. How we can go on a long break from our jobs, that it is going so well for us that we can take an extended holiday whenever we need. I think Gary could do with my help at home and sure look Mam I know you're doing great but what kind of a daughter would I be if I didn't spend time with you while you're in hospital? We might even come for Christmas. We can go straight back to Oz once you are back on your feet and out of this place, I tell her.

I don't know why I am even going back. Kieran can surely pack my things and ship them over before he gets on a plane; I can email my resignation. What if she dies while I am over there? What if I get a phone call to say it is time while I am on a plane? I will have to turn my phone off until we arrive at our layover and might find out my mother is dead while I am standing in a random airport in the Middle East. I say all of this repeatedly to my dad as we drive to Dublin airport. I say it again as he walks me to departures.

'It will be fine. She'll be here for a good while yet. These kinds of things can go on for a very long time.' I look back at him before I disappear through to security. He smiles and waves.

Freddie: *Good guy, Tony, deluded as ever.*

I take a moment during my layover in Dubai, as I sit on the metro, to remind myself that four years ago I couldn't get on the train to Dublin by myself because my psychosis had me believe I was in danger. No one trusted me to get myself from A to B. Someone had to assist me everywhere I went in case I got lost and confused or had a panic attack. It is these kinds of achievements that show me how far I have come. I hope moving back home does not erase the progress I have made.

We stay in Sydney for three more weeks, most of the time spent trying to get back home. My dad refuses to believe I should be in any rush; she will be here until March, he insists. I have to literally scream down the phone that I don't need to be a doctor to tell you she won't even see the new year. I don't know why I am looking for his permission in the first place. The man is clearly not in his right mind and in denial about losing his wife. Booking flights in December is a nightmare, as is breaking our lease and leaving our apartment. It is all a nightmare, quitting our jobs, saying goodbye to our friends and packing our things, half of which has to be thrown out because there is just no time to do it all properly.

My head swims when I get a phone call from a recruitment agent the day before we leave on behalf of a cosmetics brand that I once worked for in Ireland. The company is now in Australia and wants to offer me a long-term contract with the strong possibility of sponsoring my resident's visa if I can start right away. I see my lifelong dream float away as I say no.

We give the keys to a couple from Mayo who are moving in to our home as we move out. Our flight is not for hours so we sit on a bench and say nothing. I cannot speak, there is a physical ache in my chest as the taxi pulls up to take us away. I know I shouldn't but I look out the window while the plane takes off and get one last glimpse of the Sydney skyline as we whizz down the runway and then there is nothing but clouds. Kieran turns to look at me sadly. I don't know when I started but I am crying. 'And that's all she wrote,' he says. I nod. It is over and there is no point in pretending otherwise.

***

Saying goodbye is never easy. I have never been able to choose which I think is worse – when someone dies suddenly or when it is a long, slow goodbye. I don't think anyone can choose. The shock is the worst with the former, the other is drawn out and painful. I never imagined this sort of goodbye, though. We know she is going to die; we know the end is looming, but Mam thinks she has all the time in the world. She must know deep down. It would be incredibly selfish to expect her to acknowledge it on our behalf. There is no other choice but to have this one-sided goodbye.

She is delighted to see me back so soon; her mind is too muddled to make the connection with what this means. I tell her we're home for Christmas. In fairness, I could tell her anything at this stage and she would believe it. She tells Kieran about her plans to go shopping in New York. Everyone else has been saying goodbye for months now. I feel a surge of anger whenever I think of this. All the lies stole precious time I could have spent with her.

We try to make up for it. She has a random desire to go

for lunch with me in this hotel, something we had talked about before I left and never got to do. On the way there we have to stop at a bridal shop for a family member who wants to show Mam her dress and get a picture together. I am happy for Mam, getting to have that special moment with someone she loves. If she was in her right mind, she would know it was her only chance to see it.

It is unfortunate that I have to be there. It's nobody's fault, just the way it works out with the wheelchair taxi, that the two events have to happen together. I sit outside and it physically hurts, like someone has ripped my heart out, knowing I will never have this moment with her. When Mam comes out of the store, she sees me upset and misinterprets the reason. 'Don't worry, you'll have your day when we go and pick out your wedding dress.'

Her next random request is a trip to Cork. There are weather warnings all across the country and Teresa Mannion is shouting at everyone to not make any unnecessary journeys. Mam is determined, though; no one can look at her sad face when we try to explain it may not happen. So, we load into our rented minibus and head off. We wheel her around Brown Thomas and she buys endless amounts of skincare and make-up. Buying things seems to distract her. We finally get her out, laden down with bags full of cosmetics. When we get back to the hospice, I help her go through them.

'I have enough here to do me for the rest of my life,' she says.

Freddie: *Well, she's not wrong there.*

I wish we could acknowledge what is about to happen. When she sits up in bed, making plans for the future, I just want to scream that none of these things are going to happen. I don't want to talk to her about holidays she will never go on. I want to say goodbye, to ask her what I am supposed to do without her. She doesn't look like my mam and she doesn't sound like her. When I look at her all I see is a pretend person drowning in denial who is planning what to wear to family weddings she will never attend, memories of which she won't be part. I don't want this strange woman; I want my mam.

Freddie: *She's already gone. Like it or not, kid, this is what you got now. Make the most of what's left of her while you still can.*

I snap out of these selfish moments and remind myself that this is her way of coping. Would I rather she be sad? At least her last days are filled with laughter and happiness; she doesn't need to see our tears. All she asks of us is to pretend with her and we can do that, surely; after all, she has put on a brave face for us enough times. Louise, Jamie's fiancée, points out to me how happy she is: 'She's in a little bubble and who are we to burst it?', which is a nice way to put it.

***

I am on my own with her. She drifts in and out of sleep. She has had a bad couple of days. She seems annoyed with me;

she thinks her mother is sick and we are keeping it from her. She tells me to stop lying and tell her the truth. 'I have a right to know, I can handle it,' she shouts. Her mother is fine. Nana was only here visiting the other day. She should be down again soon for Christmas.

We were planning on bringing Mam home on Christmas Day. With enough equipment, it's possible. It is not looking likely now, though, with the way she has been, but the nurses, angels that they are, have suggested setting up a mini-Christmas dinner in the family room for us. All our family are going to travel down for it. We have never spent a Christmas with all of us together.

I get her to calm down and believe that Nana is alright. She goes back to sleep but gives me a fright when her eyes fly open and she looks frantic. 'We have to get the Christmas presents for the kids,' she tells the ceiling. 'I've hidden the Santa presents; I'll go get them.' She thinks we're in Athlone, that Jamie and I are small. She asks me to go down to John and Phyllis' house and get our presents.

Freddie: *Fuck it. Just go along with it.*

I tell her I will and she can even tell me exactly where to find them. Then she thinks she is a child and she's sitting on a wall waiting for her dad to come home from work. She wants to get her bike and tries to throw herself out of the bed. I ring the alarm at this point. She becomes hysterical, going back further in time in her head.

I escape outside when the nurses come. I make the calls, I ring everyone – my dad, Jamie, Sylvia, Mam's sisters, I don't want to misread this and worry everyone needlessly but I know it is that time, the end.

They move her next door, to the bigger room with a kitchen and toilet off to the side. There is a couch and room for a large group of people. They put this picture of a symbol of the circle of life on the door. Your loved ones can gather here and the sign tells everyone to be quiet when they pass, this is the room where people die.

Everyone makes it down from all corners of the country. We pull up chairs, drink tea and try to console each other. There is one person missing, though. Gary.

I asked earlier on that someone else tell him but everyone is busy and we ran out of time. I have to do it. It takes me a full day to find him and when I do, it is hard to come up with the right words to say. I have the worst conversation I have ever had with anyone.

When I bring him in to the hospice, he takes one look at her and storms out of the room. He breaks something off the wall in the kitchen area and we half-wrestle him onto the couch and try to get him to be quiet.

Gary has been dealing with his own issues. He was left to his own devices while I was away. All the attention has been on Mam and because he did not have enough support, his friends have become his family. No one ever knows what to do with him. I am usually the best with him but even I am at a loss. He cannot grasp that she is really going, that his mother is leaving him and he has run out of time to make things right. He gets in these frantic states where nothing can calm him down except his prescription medication, which makes him really drowsy until he falls asleep for a couple of hours. However, when he wakes up it does not take long before he turns into something like a feral animal again. The Gary we love is still in there, though; you can see it when he sits rubbing Mam's head and holding her hand or when he sits with Nana, making sure she has everything she needs, fussing over whether she is comfortable and serving her up her dinner.

He starts getting desperate for a fix as time passes. He keeps telling me and I ask him what he expects me to do about it. I don't have a dealer on speed dial. We have a family meeting out in the corridor about something or other. Gary hops up and down interjecting every few seconds that he needs *something*. Dad tells him he will go out and get him his medication. 'No, don't put me to sleep, Dad,' he shouts. A woman passing by looks very worried about what's going on here. As serious as the situation is, myself and Jamie nearly choke with laughter over how bad it looks. We are not laughing the next day as Jamie hands over a wad of cash to keep people to whom Gary owes money off his back. I sit in my car at the top of an alleyway while my little brother buys drugs. I know we might sound like terrible enablers, but right now Mam is our focus. Gary's growing problem can wait.

***

More people arrive as the days go on. Her friends file in to say their goodbyes. I go out sometimes. Kieran and I drive around in circles, looking at the lights, watching people run around doing their shopping. I scroll through social media looking at all the pictures from people's festive drinks. I see a news article about someone who died in an accident. I think of their family losing them so close to Christmas.

Freddie: *Think about that for a second.*

Oh, yeah. That's us now, we are those people that someone is going to feel sorry for. Her anniversary is going to be this time of year.

She slips in and out of consciousness. One day I hug her and she moves her head to cuddle into my shoulder; somehow, I know it is the last hug I will ever get. Another night I kiss her on the head as I am leaving. Her eyes are closed, she seems asleep. 'Love you,' she whispers and I know it is the last time I will hear her say it.

Watching someone die makes you count all the last times, trying to record them in your head. It makes you more aware of time too. Every second that ticks by brings you closer to the end and those seconds go by too fast.

She opens her eyes and smiles at whoever is around her. We all stand or sit by the bed; Kieran hovers in the background out of her sight. She always called him by his nickname. She looks around at us all and says 'Where's Ishy?'

It is the last time she speaks.

I sit in the chapel room on my own.

Freddie: *Turning to God in this difficult time?*

'There is no God, Freddie.'

Freddie: *It's time I told you the truth. All these years I have been testing you, my child, you are the messiah, the second coming of Christ. I am God.*

'Stop being stupid.'

Freddie: *If I was God, I would have blessed you with better eyebrows.*

'And given me special healing powers, so I could make her better.'

Freddie: *Yep. You could turn water into wine and bread into fish, it was fish wasn't it?*

'And if you were God, you could create people and let them into heaven when they die.'

Freddie: *I'd create all kinds of people. Give everyone noses for ears and give them extra arms coming out of their stomachs.*

'What would your heaven look like?'

Freddie: *Don't know what it would look like, but it would be happy and warm and no one would ever be sad.*

'Would you let me into your heaven?'

Freddie: *Fuck no, I've put up with your shit long enough.*

'Will you let my mam in though?'

Freddie: *I don't know, there was that one time I saw her kick a puppy or the time I saw her stealing from the charity box.*

'That never happened.'

Freddie: *Did too. Can't have the likes of her in heaven.*

'Can you stick around for a bit? I might need you later.'

Freddie: *Sure, kid. Can I get you anything?*

'Can you tell me a story or something?'

Freddie: *I'll tell you about the puppy kicking.*

'A story that actually happened, Freddie.'

Freddie: *I don't have many of those. How about a song instead?*

Sometimes I need a break. It's easier to listen to Freddie's nonsense than sit in that room and watch the life drain from her. Hearing voices in your head is supposed to be a bad thing. But Freddie serves as a distraction, if anything, most of the time. She is in a sort of coma now, she keeps making this awful sound, the nurses have ensured us that she can't feel any pain but I know the sound of her gasping and choking will haunt me for the rest of my life. We take turns saying goodbye. Everyone is to have their few minutes alone with her. Kieran offers to come in with me, and I surprise him, myself and Freddie when I accept. I thought I would want to be alone with her but I need him there.

Freddie: *We are right here with you, kid.*

I hold her hand and let the words come. I don't say anything beautiful or poetic like they do in the movies. 'I don't want to say goodbye but I know you have to go; you'll feel better when you do. So much better, you won't be sick any more. You can let go and I promise we'll be alright. I'll look after Gary, well, I'll try anyway, he's a stubborn shit.'

I take a picture of our hands together. I thank her for everything she did for us, for understanding, or at least always trying to. For sticking up for me when no one else would, for being my best friend, listening to me, teaching me how to see things from other people's perspectives, teaching me how to forgive, how to be strong, how to get back up when things are hard and keep fighting every day. Coldplay's Christmas song plays on a radio in the corner.

I kiss her hands and tell her I love her. I say goodbye as Kieran puts his hand on my shoulder and Freddie hums along to the song in my ear. For the final hour, it's just us, her children and her children-in-law. Kieran and I, Jamie and Louise and Gary sit with her, reminiscing, talking, laughing.

It gets late and we all go home for the night. She dies in our father's arms an hour later.

Chapter 16

The funeral director arrives at 2 a.m. He wanted to get in fast as, apparently, undertaking is a competitive industry. Must be strange having a business that relies on death. He is a kind man with a thick country accent. His sense of humour is welcome and makes the following few days a little easier.

My mam's sisters are inconsolable. They have no idea how to break the news to my Nana that her first born is gone. Dad has gone into work mode, conducting the process like a board meeting. Gary is asking me for help spelling a posthumous tribute for her on Facebook. Jamie, who has had a cold the last few days, is slumped on the floor after making the terrible mistake of drugging himself up to the gills with Night Nurse before the news broke.

The funeral director takes notes as we try to figure out how best to approach this. Mam made it so no plans were put in place, and we can't bury her where we want to because no one has bought a plot. Sylvia agrees to pick out an outfit for her. My dad, who usually does the eulogy for family funerals, decides to sit this one out. I nominate myself and wonder if I will regret it later. We tell the director that Jamie will take care of all the music, as he plays guitar in a band called Loungeroom Lizards. The man gives Jamie, who has almost begun drooling, a worried look. Flowers, readings, prayers of the faithful and the afters are discussed. We decide to wake her at the house rather than at the funeral home.

'She wanted nothing more than to go home,' Dad tells him 'it's only right that she goes there one last time.'

'She would like that,' Jamie tries to say.

Her removal will be tomorrow (or later today, whatever way you want to look at it). The funeral will take place the day before Christmas Eve. We wrap up quickly, more out of concern for Jamie's condition than anything else, and go home.

I sleep for a few hours. When I wake up, I forget for a moment, but then it hits me that she is gone. This is a feeling, I suspect, that I will experience every morning for a long time. I used to walk out of my room every day and look down the hall to see her sitting up in bed. Usually surrounded by mindfulness colouring books, angel cards and notes from her work-from-home 'business' that none of us had the heart to tell her was a pyramid scheme. I look now and see the hospital bed. Tomorrow I will look and see a coffin in that space.

Someone arrives later to take the bed away, along with the rest of the medical equipment. I go to a nail appointment I had already made because I don't know what else to do. I pick orange because it was her favourite colour.

Coffin shopping is next on the agenda. Dad, a less drowsy

Jamie and I stand in a room full of them and pick one out. We get a tour of the graveyard later on; the undertaker does his best impression of a real estate agent as he shows us the quality of the plot we have picked. 'Further down there you could have some drainage problems but this is a prime location,' he says enthusiastically before asking subtly about Dad's plans. He tells him to book a double plot.

I weave in and out of the crowds in town, trying to talk to as few people as possible. I don't mind those who want to come up to give their condolences, but the welcome home party is another issue. Kieran, who has lived here his whole life and knows half the town, keeps getting stopped by people surprised to see him in Ireland. We have only been back three weeks and most of the time has been spent at the hospital.

'Do you have to be so fucking polite all the time? Just say you can't talk right now. I swear if one more person asks what we are doing back.' I don't mean to take it out on him but it is packed and festive everywhere with what seems like the whole town rushing around getting presents. None of them know, they don't understand that she is dead and so nothing should be normal right now. The world looks just as it did before. Kieran gets his suit and I get my funeral clothes. 'Picking up some last-minute bits?' the girl at the till says to me cheerfully 'Yeah, nearly done now,' I reply.

The removal from the funeral home is family only. We walk into the room and see her laying in her coffin for the first time. My dad puts his hand over his mouth and bursts into tears, 'My lovely wife,' he says as he rushes over to give her a kiss on the forehead. Jamie turns off the mournful trad song playing on the stereo, the singer wailing, sounding like nails on a chalkboard. 'Silence is better than that shite,' he says, rolling his eyes. I can barely look at Gary – he has been in such a state and I don't know what to do for him.

We walk out to the hearse, a hand each on the coffin. It reminds me of how we carried Stephen. On the slow drive out home I watch people bless themselves as we pass. I may not be religious but it is still nice to see.

All I hear is noise in my head. The others are there but not saying anything important. Freddie hasn't even mentioned what has happened. The hearse tries to drive into our neighbour's house and Dad starts frantically beeping his horn at them. I don't think anyone could cope with the shock of a hearse with a coffin appearing on their front drive unexpectedly.

Once she is settled in her room, we arrange things properly. We light candles, place her favourite photographs around. Louise painted her nails with her favourite polish a few days ago, but I touch up her lipstick now.

I lay in bed that night and wonder when the real pain will start. This feels like it is happening to someone else. I know, though, that this part – when everyone is around and we are all together – is the easy part.

***

The wake is more like a party than anything else. The house is packed with people coming to pay their respects. Gary has a room full of friends, as does Jamie. Some of them have changed their plans for Christmas in order to be here and most stay for the night. A few of mine come and go but most of them don't turn up. I say to Kieran that I must be an awful person to have this poor a turnout.

The timer has started again, the seconds going too quickly. I stare at her face and try to memorise every inch of it before I never see her again. The rosary starts. I, ever the agnostic, stare at the floor for most of it until Jamie says something to make me laugh. I guess all the tension will do that to you.

At around 1 a.m. I finally sit down to write the eulogy. The only one left is one of Gary's friends who is off his head on something and sobbing into the coffin: 'That could be my mother one day, you know.' I can hear Jamie threatening to kick him out. I have put off writing this long enough so I drown them all out and put pen to paper. It is the easiest thing I ever write. I realise when I finish: that's what it's all about, isn't it? You should live your life in such a way that when someone sits down to write the eulogy for your funeral, they won't struggle to come up with good examples of your character. They won't have to exaggerate or glorify how good you were because you were one of the good ones.

I imagine what someone might write about me one day. I am no angel but I have put a lot of effort into raising mental health awareness, at least that's something. I think about a few people I know who may not get the same treatment. Not schoolyard bullies or disastrous friends, but really bad people whom I have come across. What a shit end to your life, some poor individual having to scramble to find a few good points about you among all your horribleness. In that moment, I forgive some people from my past that I never thought I would. I don't hate them any more, I pity them. I wonder, briefly, about the bad woman and the faceless man but then I remind myself that you cannot forgive people who are products of your imagination.

The condolences start pouring in. Some comment, some send private messages, a text or a phone call. People pay their respects at the graveside. 'I'm sorry for your loss', they say as they shake your hand.

The funeral is over. Everyone goes home. 'Let me know if we can do anything.'

It is now time for the next stage of grieving. 'I'm here if you need me', is what people say. Some people are not there when you need them, though. They disappear from your life after that. Some forever. It's strange how they say they're sorry for your loss, they're sorry for you because you have lost someone you love, but then they go and leave you too. So, effectively, you end up losing another person you loved. Now you have to try and get over them as well. The only difference is they have chosen to leave you. Those people must not have been all that sorry for your loss after all.

The first anniversary comes. 'This has been a tough year for you,' people say. The second anniversary comes and maybe some people are still there to tell you everything is going to be alright. The third anniversary comes. There's a whole lot of silence. The day is not marked in any way. It is hardly mentioned. It has been three years, three whole years since people said 'Sorry for your loss'. That's long enough now, some people think, time to start moving on. You probably have moved on a little. It's not that you don't feel the pain any more. That agonising, longing feeling still stabs you in the chest and washes over you like a wave when it hits you all of a sudden. You still feel it, often several times a day. The pain is just as bad as the day they died, you feel just as much. The only difference is you've gotten used to it. You suppose that's moving on in a way. No one says 'Sorry for your loss' any more. But it's okay for you to still feel sorry for your loss.

You are sorry for your loss every time you wake up and realise it wasn't just a bad dream. You are sorry for your loss when you pick up the phone before remembering there's no one at the other end. When you hear their song on the radio. When all you want for your birthday is a hug from them. When you wish you could still wrap that Christmas present. When you question why they were taken from you. When you stare at a photograph and feel that longing. When all the important milestones are happening in your life and they are not there to see it. When that memory still has the power to bring you to your knees. When you go to their favourite spot. When you pick up their old scarf and you could swear it still smells like them. When it's all going wrong and they are the only person you want to confide in. When you try to make peace with the fact that you will never speak to them again. Every time you think about how there are no more memories to be made.

In those moments, the amount of time that has passed is completely irrelevant. You are still sorry for your loss. When someone dies, it takes a little while for the really hard part to come. The wake and the funeral and the initial grieving period are difficult, of course. But what comes next is far worse. The really hard part is when they stay dead. If you are lucky enough to have not experienced this, please try to understand. And if you have been unfortunate enough to know exactly what I am talking about, well then, I'm sorry for your loss.

Chapter 17

On New Year's Eve, I write out a list. I feel like such a cliché with the day that's in it but my mother has just died so I think I am allowed this time. I write out what I want to happen, no, what I *know* is going to happen next.

Documentary

The Late Late Show (typical Irish, I know)

Write a book

We are finally going to get married as well, I decide, and maybe – if it is not too much to ask from the universe – I could look into becoming a journalist. All of this may seem impossible given our current situation, but I want to try this whole manifesting, law-of-attraction thing. The progress I made before Australia was good, but I need to reach a wider audience if I am going to leave any mark on how people view schizophrenia. Freddie still remains a secret at this point, as I don't know how to possibly describe his existence without adding to the stereotypical view people have of psychosis. I need to reduce the stigma around the illness, after all, and Freddie sounds far too much like a character from a badly made movie.

We are in a pretty bad place as it stands. I remember the night of the funeral, sitting on the floor beside Kieran with Dad, Jamie and Louise. The coffin was obviously gone, so it was just a big empty room. We tried to come up with some kind of plan for Christmas Day, deciding to go to Louise's family. When they left the room, Kieran and I remained on the floor. Gary had decided to drop out of school. Everyone else could return to their jobs or college. We had nothing. Less than a fiver sat in our bank account; we were broke from all the travelling home from Australia.

'Now what?' Kieran said.

Now what is right.

We have to start again. I spent years trying to get to Australia and it was all for nothing. And I am mad as hell. I am angry at my family for not telling me about Mam's worsening condition. I am angry at them for taking those months with her away from me. I am angry at her for playing God with my life and deciding for me like that. I could have gone now, afterwards, but no, the fucking positive squad convinced me to go, knowing full well there was a chance I would never see her again. There are five stages of grief and I have jumped straight into anger.

Dad later tells me that he knew that day, when we left for Oz, when I said goodbye to her, that it would be, as far as they were concerned, the last time she would see me. I try to ask what in the world they were all thinking. What was the plan?

To ring me up after she was dead and break the news with, 'Sorry we didn't tell you sooner, we all knew and spent the last few months saying goodbye but you missed it'? I never get an answer to that question.

There was the party they had for her birthday. They keep talking about how special it was that they were all together and it was like a big goodbye for her with all the people she loved. They forget that I wasn't there because I didn't know. They talk about how even some of Jamie's friends shed a tear at it. His friends knew before me. Family who only ever saw her every couple of years knew before me. The fucking postman knew before me. Gary is the only person who didn't know the full picture. And once again, I had to do the hard job with Gary and tell him what was going to happen. Because I have to do everything for him; for years I have had to treat him like he was my own child and put my own life on hold to look after him. And here I am back again, looking after him, cooking him dinners that he doesn't eat, cleaning up after him, watching his friends take over the house because since Dad went back to work it has been a free for all for Gary.

The calls keep coming, the messages; he keeps racking up debts. When these people don't get their money they go after us instead. We are exposed to a world we should have no part in. Dad bails him out. Jamie bails him out. My paranoid mind does not deal well with people threatening me but I have no choice. The guards arriving at the door becomes a regular occurrence. We're all on a first-name basis now. I spend hours at the station one night after Gary is arrested. At one point, a guard has to stand between the two of us because Gary is taking his emotions out on me. Kieran doesn't know how to help me; I am drowning in grief and anger.

Freddie: *When you gonna tell him?*

'Twelfth of never.'

Freddie: *Come on, you have to tell him sometime.*

I have been keeping a secret. I want to talk to Kieran about it. But I can't even form the words. If I say it out loud it makes it real.

Freddie: *Fine, keep it to yourself. You're good at that.*

'I'm grieving, now is not the time to be dealing with this.'

Freddie: *Wah. Wah. Wah. People's parents die all the time. At least you had a mom, some people don't even get that lucky. How long do you think you're gonna be sad for? Because it is really dragging now.*

'Stop it, Freddie, please I can't deal with you right now.'

Freddie: *Just tell him and get it over with. It might stop you from being such a bore over this dead mom thing. I want to get back to the good stuff.*

A few days after she died, I went looking through her things. I saw a box file with my name on it. There were files and letters inside. Notes, from appointments I had with psychologists. They date back to when I was really young. I read them all. I read them and then I know. There are a few different names for it, references to traumatic amnesia, repressed memories.

The bad woman and the faceless man, two people to whom I gave silly names and somewhere along the line decided were make-believe people, products of my imagination. But, as it turns out, they were real. The root of most of my problems, the reason I have schizophrenia, can be traced back to them and how, instead of dealing with the trauma, I had some kind of split from reality instead.

I am not going to go into any detail about who they are or what either of them did. This plot twist in my story is going to be pretty anticlimactic. My reaction at the time was to put the file away and pretend I didn't read it. Burying my mother was enough hardship to go through that week. I kept going back to it, though, poring over the words, desperately trying to hold onto the idea that it was all pretend, that it didn't matter.

I tell Kieran eventually; he has heard enough about these people from listening to me recount my mixed-up memories over the years. He is as shocked as I am. I talk to a few people who would know, who might fill in some of the blanks for me. I get flashbacks. My memories are like scattered jigsaw puzzles, but with every piece the overall picture starts to make sense. Looking back, I can see Mam had tried to test my memory several times, especially around the time when I was diagnosed; she wanted to see how much I remembered. I was probably better off not knowing, I would still be in the dark if I had not found the file. Maybe, one day, I will try to deal with what happened, but not now. I still like to pretend that they were never real. It makes me feel better. That may seem unhealthy to some people, it might sound like I am running away from a problem. I know I will have to face up to what happened one day. But, right now, I feel like I have had quite enough demons to deal with.

Freddie: *Some therapist is gonna have a field day with this one.*

***

I have always been a planner. I think far ahead and like to know exactly how things are going to pan out. As you may have guessed, this hasn't gone very well for me so far. But I need to do something. I start a night course in radio, just to test the waters. I don't tell the others on the course that I am grieving, so it works out as a little escape for me every week from the drama at home. The course makes me realise that I will never be content until I give journalism a go.

It is not ideal, going back to college in my late twenties, but I know it is the right thing for me. Besides, it is on the list and the list needs to happen. After losing out on my Australian dream, I need a new focus. Everything up until this point has been about moving to Oz. It is time for a new dream.

I know I have aimed high; it is all fairly unrealistic, impossible even, but one thing I have learned about myself is that I am stubborn and determined and, once I get an idea in my head, nothing can pull me back down to earth. I was once told to not expect very much from my life with my diagnosis. I believed it for a while. I thought having a mental illness meant I wouldn't ever really achieve anything. I was once told by a medical professional that people like me are not capable of much and I should aim low. But that was a load of shite. I have done fairly well, all things considered. If I want to study journalism, do a documentary, go on *The Late Late Show* and write a book then I will. I will get married and all.

I set up a few new social media accounts called Pretty Sane. I post about mental health, my life, support networks available; I talk about things that I have found helpful and all the rest. It works as an outlet for me, helps with my writing and means I'm raising awareness at the same time. I start talking to followers about their mental health and they help me as much as I help them.

A week later, out of the blue, I get an email from a producer named Aoife Kavanagh about a documentary she is researching. The subject is schizophrenia. I speak to her over the phone first. During our conversation, I mention that Mam died recently and she tells me that she has lost her mother too. 'Does it get any easier?' I ask. 'No, but the crying on the kitchen floor in the middle of the night stops eventually.' I really like her after that.

She comes to my house to do a screen test and we talk about other people who could be included in the program. We both mention Michelle from Cork. I read about her a few years ago and Brian from Wexford too. Then there is Rita, whom I have known for years through See Change. I post on social media, looking for anyone who would like to share their story.

As a society, we have this idea that schizophrenia and psychosis are rare, but let me tell you – they are not. It's just that the stigma attached to them stops people from speaking out about them. Eight people, all living within a couple of miles of my house, contact me. I live in a small town and I can think of several people, apart from those eight, who are like me. We don't get much representation in the mental health campaigns but there are plenty of us. Almost all of those people decide not to go ahead with it, as they are either too scared to let anyone know or nervous about how it might affect them in relation to employment.

With my course coming to an end, I start to think about what to do next apart from the documentary. Then, because tragedy seems to strike in pairs, my paternal grandad, John, is found dead of a suspected heart attack outside his home by Sylvia. This comes three months after we lost Mam. We say goodbye again, watch the coffin close and bury another one of us. Our numbers are dwindling and we become more divided with every passing day.

The Gary situation rages on. Jamie is busy planning his wedding and is more focused on his new family. It always seems like he prefers the family he is marrying into over us and I can't say I blame him. We are a disaster. One drama after another. We go on a family holiday but Gary gets arrested the night before we leave, which puts a dampener on things. The truth is, Mam was the glue that held us all together and, without her, we fall apart. We are all to blame in some way. My bitterness over Australia and being kept in the dark doesn't help matters. I know I need to let my anger go. I should know better than to blame my problems on other people.

Speaking of problems, my party trick is avoiding mine like the plague until it all gets too much and I have a breakdown. So, in keeping with this self-destructive pattern, I decide what better way is there to pile stress onto myself than planning a wedding. A new wedding, completely different from the one we were supposed to have before. I also decide that organising the entire thing in ten months is a wonderful idea.

When it comes to planning your wedding or any significant life event, everything can become about what should happen, how things should be, which adds an awful amount of pressure. Think about it, how many times have you found yourself unhappy with something in your life because of what you think it should be? Or ever been disappointed in someone because they are not doing what you think they should do? You think you should be more successful; you should be doing this that or the other.

HOW TO BE MENTAL TIP 21

Stop using the word 'should' when assessing your happiness. Things should be this way or that. When you learn to see past the picture of what you thought your life should look like, it makes it easier to enjoy the moment.

That tip comes from future me. Past me did not do this. She planned her wedding while drowned in grief and full of resentment.

I know my mam will always be with me. I am sure she is with me in her own special way, and that is lovely and comforting at times. But did that help when I went to dress fittings to be met with 'Oh, you've come on your own again?', or every time I had to tell a supplier that no thank you the mother of the bride would not be requiring anything, or when I had a meltdown over flowers because I know literally nothing about them and they were always her thing, or the time I cried on the floor holding the teddy that she had died beside? No, that thought didn't help at those times.

I am not good with making decisions. Now I know some brides are plagued by their mothers'/sisters'/aunts' opinions, which can be incredibly frustrating when trying to please everyone. But I have the opposite problem; I have no opinions. From colour schemes, to entertainment, to food, to accessories, all major decisions come down to me and me alone. I never have anyone to tell me 'No, that's not a good idea'. Asking someone for an opinion is always met with 'Whatever you want; it's your day' or 'You know best'. This all comes from a good place but I crave some blunt honesty. I need someone to be critical so I don't have to mull over every decision, wondering whether I have genuinely made the right choice or people are just avoiding hurting my pride.

I have developed a habit of automatically counting every mother/daughter duo I see when I walk into a restaurant or when I am out shopping. When I see mothers helping their daughters with their own children, I think how the hell will I ever manage motherhood myself without her support. I get this strange feeling when I am going somewhere that I am missing or have forgotten something and then I recognise the feeling; it is longing. That feeling is the worst, probably because it physically hurts; it's this pain you get in your chest. All you need is the person who is gone, and your heart aches for them to be there.

***

It is all a bit of a whirlwind of a year. We have family weddings on both sides, I get back to my mental health talks and events, I publish a couple of articles. I don't think, worry, analyse. I don't feel. I just do. I start college in September, and my only fellow mature student is a nice man in his seventies. I am surrounded by people who are coming straight from school. And do you know what, it's the best thing for me. Over the next few years, I have some pretty low points, and being entertained by the antics and dramas of a bunch of nineteen-year-olds is refreshing, an escape from being an adult. Plus, people of that age group are hilarious: the world hasn't crushed their spirit yet, as Freddie says.

My spirit is well and truly crushed at this stage. Things have not worked out at home. Due to what has been going on with Gary, I don't feel safe there any more. Kieran and I have been living out of a suitcase for six weeks now, which is about as fun as it sounds. Since Mam died, it has been one thing after another. I don't stop to process any of it. Our couch-sleeping days come to an end when we find somewhere to live – the same house we lived in before we moved home to save for Australia. We have come full circle, it seems.

The closer it gets to Christmas, the more dread I feel. The thought of hearing the same songs that played while we said goodbye to her, seeing those lights again. I know it is going to bring everything back. I write a piece called 'When it's not the most wonderful time of the year' for 'A Lust for Life'.

HOW TO BE MENTAL TIP 22

Here we go with the 'should' again. Certain times of the year can bring extra pressure to be happy. In the summer, you are supposed to be out having fun in the sun. Christmas should be filled with festive cheer. You are expected to enjoy all of your birthdays. Life is too messy and complicated to guarantee the idea of significant events being perfect or always going to plan. Bad shit happens regardless of the time of year.

We try to make the most of it, though. Jamie and Louise get married in December. We get through the anniversary and Christmas itself. I don't burst into tears as the clock strikes twelve on New Year's as I did the year before. It has been the toughest year so far, but I got through it. I may have spent most of it in a dissociated state, going through the motions but I did the best I could. I survived.

Filming for the documentary starts up, which gives me something positive to focus on. There are six of us taking part. Michelle has heard voices since she was a child and, like me, has gotten used to them and accepted them to the point that she doesn't want them to go away. She rejects the term schizophrenia and prefers to use the term voice hearer. Then there is Alex. His psychosis came on suddenly when he was a teenager. He went to a concert and nothing was amiss until he came home and asked his mother, 'Do you realise I'm the anti-Christ?' Alex said he went into a deep sleep, dreamt he was being chased by the devil and felt a burning sensation. He spent the following years in and out of hospital, believing he was a descendant of Abraham, here to make peace on Earth. Like me and my mind reading, my inanimate objects and my crows, he believes these things because, to us, they are real. As Michelle puts it when it comes to voices, 'This idea that you shouldn't listen to voices because they are not real. Bullshit. Just because you can't hear them doesn't mean they're not real. I can hear them so they're real to me.'

A psychologist, who is interviewed as part of the documentary, talks about how the attitude towards psychosis is changing. We used to be told not to listen to the voices, but now we are encouraged to listen to them. In the hospital, they would tell me to listen to them for a short while once a day. Freddie thought this was the funniest thing he ever heard. I do practise it, though. I only acknowledge Freddie when I want to, unless he is being particularly persistent. It works better with the other voices and sounds; I wouldn't say I can control them, but I do have a choice in how much attention I pay them. I'm one of the lucky ones, as I can drown them out and I can talk myself out of a delusion.

Brian is not as lucky. Like me, he uses music to drown out the voices. It is the delusions he struggles with; he gets paranoid when people use certain words. Simple words and everyday phrases trigger his delusions, like 'perfect', 'absolutely', 'exactly', 'indeed', 'sure', 'oh my God', 'definitely', 'certainly', 'how's it going', 'how are things', 'how you getting on', 'hmm', 'spot on', 'of course', 'fair play' and 'best of luck'.

Or when people clear their throat or put their hair behind their ears. He thinks these words and actions are directed specifically towards him to make him paranoid. He believes people on the radio and television are trying to send him messages. Like in Alex's case, his psychosis began suddenly.

Bethany, who is nineteen, has heard voices for most of her life but a year ago they took a more sinister turn and began telling her to kill herself. Her dad also has schizophrenia, which he says is like a living nightmare. His voices scream at him all day; the only break he gets is when he goes to sleep at night. Rita also takes part; her illness is different from what the rest of us have, as she experiences the negative symptoms. (Negative symptoms can be anything from social withdrawal to decreased motivation.)

The documentary is expected to air on RTÉ later in the year. Speaking of RTÉ, while we are filming, the station airs another documentary, *Medication Nation*, presented by Dr Eva Orsmond. If you haven't heard of Dr Eva, she is a Finnish doctor and weight-loss expert who appears on a lot of Irish reality shows, such as *Operation Transformation*, *Dancing with the Stars*, that kind of stuff. Her documentary is about the overuse of prescription medication. The discussion around antidepressants and anti-anxiety dugs raises some controversy. I am asked to write a piece on it for *The Journal*. I write about the good and the bad, how I think it is important to highlight how destructive addiction to over-the-counter and prescription medication can be. On the other side, I talk about how I felt that the programme came across as being dismissive towards medication for mental health. I make the point that a person who is too mentally unwell to get out of bed can struggle to participate in the more active side of self-care, like exercise. Medication can be the driving force behind what gets a person up in the morning so that they can bring the dog for a walk, cook a healthy meal or participate in therapy. Medication is not a crutch but can be a helping hand towards stability.

I also point out how there is a huge stigma surrounding mental health problems, therefore I do not agree with anything that encourages this and creates a sense of shame around taking medication to help with an illness. In the mental health community, there has always been a bit of a debate between people who are pro-medication and anti-medication. I fall somewhere in the middle. I don't take medication myself any more, but if someone was to present me with a drug that cured my mental health problems, of course I would try it. However, since medication doesn't work for me, I appear like someone on the anti-medication side, which I'm not.

When the article comes out, the headline (which is not written by me) is 'I live with schizophrenia without taking any medication, but I'm an exception'. Cue my very first experience with trolls and hate online.

Some people jump on the headline without reading the piece itself and think that my not taking medication must mean I am against it. Then I have people who say a schizophrenic not on medication is dangerous and encourages others to stop taking theirs, that I should be locked up, that people like me are a danger to society, what if I hurt someone, and so on.

The thought of being trolled had always terrified me since speaking publicly about my illness. But when it actually happens, it is not so bad at all, as for every negative message or comment, there is a positive one. I find them funny for the most part. My hen is the weekend after and we have a little fun with it, dressing up like criminals in orange jumpsuits with a sign that says 'Danger to Society'.

This incident is the first of many, but I don't mind it for the most part. The negative ones only serve as a reminder of how far we have to go in ending mental health stigma. Every time I think I have raised enough awareness for schizophrenia and it might be time to give it a rest, a throwaway account with a fake profile picture calls me a schizo and gives me motivation to keep going.

Chapter 18

With the wedding around the corner, I have never been so stressed. Despite Kieran's initial protest, it has a Harry Potter theme – a classy version, not the 'kids party people dressing up as wizards' type. This is what I tell myself as I try to turn Ferrero Rochers into golden snitches while deciding whether my grandaunt should sit at the table called 'Everyday I'm muggling' or if she would prefer 'I got ninety-nine problems but a snitch ain't one'.

One of Mam's friends does all the flowers while another gets the cake. It is incredibly kind of them to do such nice things for me, even though she is gone. It means a lot to me. I plan most of the wedding by myself and it is by far the loneliest thing I have ever done. While I walk around Penney's picking out decorations I see a mother and daughter who are doing the same thing. I try very hard to get away from them, but every time I move away they seem to appear beside moments later. The mother picks up various candles and the daughter either agrees they would go nicely or tuts at her that they don't go with her rustic theme. I wish I had a mam to tut at. Although, if she were here, I would never get away with associating my nuptials with a series of fantasy novels about a boy wizard. A week before the wedding, I accidentally pretend Mam is alive. In my defence, I don't do it on purpose. I am at a salon and the beauty therapist is one of those people who cause you to struggle to get a word in. As soon as I tell her I am getting married she launches into a speech about everything wedding related. She talks about every wedding she has ever been at, what she liked, didn't like.

'Make sure you leave plenty of time for the getting ready in the morning, go through all the locations for the photographs in advance, you don't want to be flapping around on the day looking for a place with a nice backdrop. Oh and get the hotel to keep the flowers cool the night before.'

Freddie: *I am getting real tired of all this wedding shit.*

'Not long to go, Freddie, it will all be over soon.'

Freddie: *You talking about the big day or this woman's monologue?*

'She actually has some good tips.'

Freddie: *You're not even listening, she just asked you a question.*

'Sorry, what was that?'

'I said, have you checked with everyone that they're not going to wear white on the day? You can never be too careful; all it takes is one attention-seeking so and so wanting to steal the limelight.'

'I'm not sure I want the limelight.'

'But it's your day. It's all about you. And trust me, it goes by in the blink of an eye. One minute you're sipping Prosecco for breakfast and the next you're saying the goodbyes at the end of the night. It goes by in a blur, appreciate every moment. They always say you should have some alone time with your husband on the day, be sure to do that, but I'll give you a good one, in the morning when you're in the dress and ready to go, the most important thing of all is you have some time alone with your mother.'

Freddie laughs.

Freddie: *Oh shit.*

'Just the two of you, mother and daughter. Because yes, it is your day but the only other person who has looked forward to it as much is your mother. Take ten minutes alone with her because you won't ever have that time again and no one will ever be able to settle your nerves better than a mother. And you are her baby, she will want that time with you before you get swept up in the madness of the day.'

Freddie: *Please. Please. Please tell her. It will be the funniest thing. She'll die.*

I nod at her. She's still going. 'Don't forget how special this day is for her, after all this is the only time she is going to be the mother of the bride.'

I curse myself for telling her earlier that I only have brothers when she asked about my friends being bridesmaids. I need to tune her out.

'Freddie, can you distract me please?'

Freddie: …

'Say something.'

Freddie: *Nah this is too funny.*

'Make sure she's involved in everything; I know mothers can be a bit much and she is probably annoying you but her opinion is the most important of all. She must be so looking forward to it, is she?'

'Yep,' I say after a pause.

'Did she get her outfit yet?'

'She did.'

'Where did she get it?'

'Oasis.'

I am committed then. My fictional mother gets a fascinator from Debenhams because she felt a hat was too much. She's getting the hair and make-up done with myself and the bridesmaids. She didn't go on the hen because it wasn't her scene so we went on a spa weekend instead. She is very excited for the big day and she got her shoes in Brown Thomas, said she would splash out for the occasion.

Freddie: *Wow.*

I can't tell the poor woman, not after she has spent a solid ten minutes talking about the importance of a mother on your wedding day. I have no regrets, I actually enjoyed pretending to have a mam for those few minutes. And besides, you don't want to upset someone when they're in the middle of waxing you.

***

One o'clock in the morning the night before the wedding.

Okay, not bad. I have to be up at eight. Tonight, of all nights, I need to sleep. I am on my lonesome in the honeymoon suite.

Kieran left an hour ago. I nearly cried, for some reason, saying goodbye to him.

'What are you getting upset for? I'll see you tomorrow,' he said.

I told him I didn't know but could he do the big emotional goodbye with me anyway. We made that stupid 'See you at the top of the aisle' 'I'll be the one in the white' joke and then he was gone and I was alone. I had no idea what had gotten into me, I loved being alone. I should have been happy about being able to starfish on the bed while he had to go bunk in with one of the groomsmen. I could hear Kieran running back up the stairs. He must have decided he couldn't stand to spend a night without me, 'Fuck tradition,' he would say and swoop me up into his arms.

'I forgot my charger,' he said instead and exited again with a quick goodbye.

'Wait,' I shouted down the stairs at him. He took one look at my face and came back to the room.

I tried to do this thing I learned in therapy where you try to identify what exactly is causing your anxiety. I was worried that I wouldn't sleep, I was worried that I would be in the bad place the following day and I was worried something was going to go wrong. There I did it. I identified the problem, acknowledged my feelings and spoke about them to someone. It wasn't that hard. Kieran gave me a pep talk and I said goodbye to him, this time feeling much better.

And now it's one o'clock and I am still awake but it is okay because I am going to fall asleep soon, I am going to wake up in the good place and everything is going to go right. And that is the last thought I have before I go to sleep.

It's dark when I wake up. 5 a.m. I count back. Four hours. Okay, not ideal, but it could have been worse. Then it comes. The big wave washes over me and I am there, in the bad place.

The voices are loud, the noises are loud and even my own inner voice is negative. I feel sad, I wish my mam was here, I am nervous, anxious and so many people have left me down by not being there for me in the run up to this. Everything is awful.

I try to shake it off as the morning goes by, breakfast with my bridesmaids, hair and make-up, photos, they all happen around me but I am not there. Physically maybe yes, but my mind is like mud, my thoughts are surrounded by the fog. I am in full dissociation mode but I cannot let it show. If I give into this there will be no going back. The crew for the documentary arrives and I smile through my interview. If I am honest about how I am feeling I will have to acknowledge the state of my mental–health.

I can hardly breathe by the time I am at the bottom of the aisle. We are getting married in a theatre that is part of the hotel. Neither of us is religious, so it makes more sense. I will have to walk down a couple of steps and hope I don't fall; once I am down those, I can properly see every pair of eyes on me and I want the ground to swallow me up.

Stop looking. Stop looking. Stop looking.

I should have gone with my original idea and eloped. I am supposed to say here that as soon as I see Kieran it all goes away. I see the love of my life, the darkness lifts and I remember why this day is special, but that is some fairy tale bullshit. In reality, I trip over my dress and do a barely noticeable stumble before righting myself. I stand awkwardly not knowing what to do with myself while my dad gives Kieran a hug. Kieran turns to me then, gives me a kiss on the forehead, and we sit down.

'You look unreal,' he says like a fourteen-year-old trying to get the shift at an underage disco.

'I think you're supposed to say something more romantic, like beautiful,' I whisper back.

He shrugs and I smile back at him.

The officiant starts talking then and so does Freddie.

Being a non-religious ceremony, it is short, about twenty minutes. Freddie has decided to make it his mission to get me to laugh before it is over. I only barely hold it together while he does his running commentary. Out of sheer nerves, Kieran doesn't look at me but at the officiant while he says his vows. He stares at her intently while he repeats after her.

'I take thee Nicola, to be my lawfully wedded wife ...'

Freddie: *Is he marrying you or her?*

My shoulders start shaking, I put my hand over my mouth trying to keep it in but between Kieran, Freddie and all the tension I am feeling it is no use. I absolutely lose it in peals of hysterical laughter in front of everyone.

By the time I recover, Kieran is also laughing with me and I feel sheer relief. Everything is fine, almost everyone in this room loves us and we are finally becoming husband and wife. Fuck the bad place, I refuse to spend one of the biggest days of my life there.

It is not until the next day, when it is just the two of us, laughing again at some stupid running joke in the wedding party group chat, that it really hits me that we are married. Things went a bit pear shaped on our wedding day. We spent too much time focusing on making the guests happy instead of ourselves, all while both little and big things went wrong throughout the day, and the whole affair ended in a family row over some drama. But there were good things too, we had fun with the people who truly matter. We couldn't have asked for better bridesmaids and groomsmen and, most importantly, we became husband and wife. On our nine-year anniversary, I married my favourite person and my best friend. The person who went to the other side of the world because I wanted to, the person who has stuck by me through everything, the person who spent seven hours on public transport to sit in a psychiatric hospital with me for half an hour. Some people spend their whole lives searching for their person and I found mine when I was a teenager. Three weeks after I tried to end it all. If I had succeeded in that overdose, Kieran and I would have never gotten together.

HOW TO BE MENTAL TIP 23

I wish someone had told me this when I thought that there was no other way out of the darkness. I look back on every time I contemplated suicide, every time I used a knife or took an overdose or stood on the edge of the cliff and think about how far I have come since each of those times. I could have died and never known how it would all pan out. Don't end your journey, stay alive and give yourself a chance to experience what is ahead.

Chapter 19

After I get married, after I finish my exams for the summer, when the documentary is all but finished filming, it starts. For the first time since Mam died, I don't have any major projects on, the family drama has simmered down a bit and life is somewhat quiet. I don't like when it is quiet. I may not have much experience with silence but I know what quiet is. Quiet is when I have nothing but my own mind, and my mind is known to be a dangerous place when it is given free rein to do what it wants.

I could be cooking, watching television, walking down the street when it happens, there is no warning, no ominous signs.

It's sad she won't ever see her son get married but what can we do. On some beach in Bondi while her mother's dying. She's going to die soon, don't ask me how I know I just do, I need to come home now I never should have come back, will you please listen to me? All you care about is drugs when your mother is going to die. I don't know what it is, I just get the feeling this is it everyone needs be to here as soon as possible this is the end. I found something, in my mam's room, they weren't in my head, they were real. Could you come down to the station we have your brother. I have to get three grand today or I'm fucking dead. We thought you didn't remember. I need my money or I'm coming to your house, choice is yours.

I cannot blame the voices this time; it's not them. There are memories but I am not thinking of them, I am reliving them. The flashbacks keep happening and I don't know how to make them stop. I don't see them in my head, I see them, feel them, smell them, as if I have been thrown into a time machine, forced to experience the worst moments of my life multiple times a day. It goes from recent events to way back when I was a child. I know from Gary what PTSD is. I know what is happening and I understand I did this to myself. I am such a hypocrite, telling people to look after their mental health when I have ignored my own issues until they became this. This is entirely new and I am way out of my depth.

I am not strong enough for this, I have so much going on right now, I cannot handle another thing. If I actually did something wrong, I could handle it, but I didn't do it, I don't know why anyone would make this up. Why can't you call her and ask her? I have witnesses, they know I didn't do it; they were all there, ask them.

Oh, I know this one.

They don't believe me and I don't know who to go to. No, Mam, I'm so fucking sorry but I have to do this I can't take any more.

Freddie: *Ah that's the time when that woman made up that thing about you in work and there was a whole investigation but you nearly didn't get your name cleared because you decided to go down to the road and throw yourself in front a car, being dramatic as fuck until your mom stopped you?*

'Yeah, that's the one.'

Freddie: *What a ride that was.*

Then my hair falls out. I wake up one morning and feel a bald patch. I look in the mirror, using my phone to see the back and it has come out in chunks, there are patches of missing hair all over my scalp. I sit on the couch crying while Kieran inspects the damage. 'No, nothing. I swear, I wouldn't lie to you. There are no bald patches, it's all there,' he says in a serious tone, knowing it is best not to laugh, and get me more worked up. I look again and I can still see them. 'If your hair was falling out, you would see it all over the place,' he looks around 'there's none.' This means I can add delusions and hallucinations onto the list as well as the PTSD symptoms.

Another day, I walk out of the kitchen and see Kieran going up the stairs, but when I enter the sitting room, he is also there. There are two of him. Kieran number two is on the phone and speaking normally. When I go upstairs to find Kieran number one, he is gone. Therefore, Kieran number two is Kieran number one, the real Kieran, and this is getting much worse.

I decide the outside world is no longer safe and I don't want to leave the house any more. I spend as much time at home as possible. Kieran goes to work and I stay at home, worrying about alien invasions. Every now and again something unavoidable comes up and we stand at the door while Kieran gently coaxes me out like a frightened animal. I hate every second I am outside; my anxiety is through the roof and I feel as though everyone is watching me. My mind seems to be in a constant state of depersonalisation. I am in a dream, none of this is real. My life doesn't seem real and neither do I. I stare at a hand or a leg and think 'It's not real, it's not mine, I'm in a dream and I can't wake up'.

Everything is too much and I cannot stand it any longer. We cancel our honeymoon and I feel shit about it.

I start to form a plan, a fool-proof way of ending my life. I am not going to fail this time. I know I am selfish, doing this to Kieran when we have only gotten married. I know he needs me as much as I need him but I don't feel like I have a choice. I need to silence these inner demons once and for all; they are going to kill me anyway. I might as well do it now and take some control over the situation.

Surprisingly, I haven't self-harmed this time. The last time I did was my birthday last year when I had an argument with a friend. A stupid reason but Kieran went into a shop and left me in the car. He had been stuck to my side all day because it was my first birthday without Mam and I was upset in general. I started looking for something as soon as he got out of the car. It was the middle of the day with people walking past constantly so I had to be discreet. I broke up a coke can, one of my old methods for when my parents would lock all the sharp objects away. I rolled up my sleeve and went to town.

Kieran got a little mad when he found out later but bandaged me up and made me swear not to do it again. For once, I have kept that promise. Until now, at least, when I am very much about to break it. I don't particularly want to die but I don't want to live like this either.

I decide I am going to do it away from home. The people who own the house are nice and I worry that they might have trouble selling it if I were to go and die in it. There is no specific plan of when I am going to go. I will stay as long as I possibly can.

I'm happy Kieran's going to Australia; I'm just sorry he's stuck with a cunt like you. You know why you cut yourself? Because you're a schizophrenic. It's not my fault. You can't blame other people for you being a schizo. Your girlfriend is a liar. I can't wait until you find out what she's really like. I'm going to laugh and you're going to cry. Bitch. Bitch. Bitch. Not everything is about you. When I asked you what you do when you are stressed you held your arm up like it was some kind of trophy. Like you were proud of it. Harming yourself is serious, it is what people who are mentally unwell do. It is not something you do for attention. People like you go nowhere in life. You'll be in the queue for the social welfare and a council house if you keep going the way you're going. Stupid, foolish bitch. Waste of space. You're never going to do anything with your life. You remember what I told you? You don't be talking. Bad things happen to silly girls who talk. Do you not think you were asking for it? I know you want it. Come on. Stop fighting and take it. Turn and face the wall. It won't take long. It will be over soon.

'I can't do it. I can't do it, Freddie,' I gasp, struggling to breathe.

Freddie: *Yes, you can. You can do anything. Stop this shit right now and we can all go on and put this behind us.*

'No, you don't understand.'

Freddie: *Of course I do, I understand everything about you. And I know you're fucking mental and annoying and a drama queen and fuck up all the time but you're a good person. You think kindly about people even when you don't like them or if they do fucked up shit to you. I know your thoughts; I hear them and they're good. You're a good person and you've got your whole life ahead of you to keep doing stupid things but it all works out okay in the end anyway.*

'It keeps happening. It keeps going bad. I get on track and then it falls apart again.'

Freddie: *I'm not letting you do this.*

'You can't stop me, you're not even real.'

We go back and forth until the woman with the posh British accent intervenes.

'*Nicola was such a kind soul. She lit up every room she entered. We all loved her dearly. She was a terribly troubled young lady who fought as hard as she could until she reached such a tragic end. We wish the poor thing reached out; we would have dropped everything in a heartbeat to be by her side. If only she tried to seek help.*'

That stops me in my tracks.

Freddie: *You hearing what I'm hearing? That's what they'd say about you, kid. A load of bullshit about how you were this and that. Acting like they never ignored you when you asked for help. Mourning at your funeral, putting stuff on social media like they gave a shit. The ones who never talked to you about your illness, who refuse to believe it's even there. The ones that only think to contact you every now and again, feeling good about themselves when they throw you some attention like you're some sort of charity case or something.*

I don't think of a response but he can hear me mulling it over and my mood changing. There is nothing that drives me away from suicide more than the thought of people feeling sorry for me, pitying me, and of the ones who were never there acting like my death has an impact on them. I never want to die being remembered as 'the poor girl with the mental problems'. I am much more than that.

Freddie: *You get me?*

I nod. I have no idea if he can see it.

Freddie: *Okay, now put the bleach away and let's carry on with our day. Nothing to see here.*

I panic for a bit about who to turn to for help. I don't think any kind of health insurance would cover another hospital stay. There is another hospital to which I have never been before; I met the consultant who specialises in psychosis there when we were being interviewed on a show together. That place probably won't be an option, though, as I can't afford it. I am not sure if I even need to go to hospital, this might pass soon.

Maybe it is because I have spent the last few months being open and honest about my psychosis with Aoife and the director of the documentary, Kim, but they are the ones to whom I end up going to for help. Aoife finds me a counsellor. At our first appointment I ask would he mind if we skip the cognitive behavioural therapy or any other kind of method, apart from talking. Because that is all I want to do, I don't want to assess the why, who or how, I don't want homework, exercises or to understand how my thoughts, feelings and behaviour impact me. I want to talk until I have let every bad thought out of my brain to someone other than Kieran who has heard it all before.

I tried many types of therapy over the years and plain old talking is the one I struggle with the most, from sitting mute in front of professionals as a child, to doing the same thing while a doctor tells me I am looking for attention. But I am not scared of talking any more. I talk about everything, how I miss my mother, my family. I talk about all the things I don't understand; I know how to make friends but I don't get how to keep them. I don't know how to be myself, to stop trying to please everyone, why I find the simplest of tasks difficult. I help other people with their mental health but I never know how to apply the same methods to myself. I hate the way I look along with many aspects of my personality. My temper gets the better of me, I can be bitter, hypocritical and too hard on people. I am still sad I missed out on so much of my childhood because of learning difficulties and psychosis. I am still angry about Australia and not being told what was happening at home. I lost years of my life to mental illness. I should have made better choices; I could have done better. Friends and family walk out of my life all the time and I can never shake the feeling that it is because I am not good enough.

He is one of the good ones. He listens and understands. I bounce back from this period of ill mental health faster than ever before. I like to refer to that breakdown as to an aftershock, as I felt the effects of all the bad things that had happened to me and started to accept that most of those situations were out of my control.

HOW TO BE MENTAL TIP 24

You cannot run from trauma forever. Talking about it gives you the opportunity to make peace with whatever happened to you. Forgive yourself for making the best possible choices you could make at the time. Go easy on yourself for not having all the answers, no one does after all. Be gentle with yourself for your faults and allow others to have theirs. Forgive yourself for doing whatever is you had to do to survive.

Chapter 20

I am on the other side of the aftershock. I am doing better, much better. Back in college and counting down the days until the documentary comes out. I am nervous but at the same time I am so ready for people to see our world.

Brian, Michelle, Alex, Bethany, Rita and I, we have all suffered under the weight of the stigma attached to our illness. The reason I started advocating for schizophrenia in the first place is that I wanted people to see and understand that we're not something from a horror movie or a sensationalist headline. That is not to say that I am not freaking out inside about some of what people are about to see. When I was in the bad place, my aftershock, we shot a scene of me at one of my worst times. Kim came alone with just a camera and sat across from me while I cried about the voices in my head and had a little rant about my hand not being real. There was no pressure to do it, I wanted to. I knew the documentary would contain me talking about how far I have come, about being off medication and my wedding day. I didn't want anyone who has psychosis to sit at home watching it wondering why they are still in the bad place while I'm off living a normal life. Kim put the idea to me and reassured me that it was more than okay to say no, but I wanted to show the other side too, how bad I can get.

The documentary airs on 19 September 2017. The reception is amazing. It does everything I hoped it would. It sparks a conversation, gets people talking about schizophrenia, and the feedback is lovely. I scroll through comments and messages, feeling particularly pleased when others with schizophrenia say they felt represented and when people say the show helped them to understand a loved one's illness better.

A week later the documentary features on *Gogglebox* and I watch people watch my story. They have condensed it down to just my story, which I am not prepared for. I can barely watch and hold my breath for what feels like the whole thing as people sit on their couches and say things like, 'You'd never think there was anything wrong with her.' When I say something about being told to keep my diagnosis a secret after I was first diagnosed, someone says, 'Sweep it under the carpet, good old Ireland'. They ooh and aah at my wedding and my stomach drops once they get to the bit of me crying on my couch. Someone says I look like a different person compared to what they have seen so far. What surprises me is how fascinated they are about the voices. Seeing people shocked at something that is the most normal thing in the world to me is strange. After all these years, I still cannot get my head around how other people don't hear them, how they don't have a Freddie. I struggle to comprehend how quiet their minds must be with only their own thoughts.

Another week later and Aoife rings me in the late afternoon to ask if I would like to appear on *The Late Late Show*. Which is fixed for tomorrow night. I just about die before saying yes because I might never get this opportunity again. We wanted to spread awareness for schizophrenia, after all, and there is not a bigger platform in Ireland to do so.

After a mad twenty-four hours during which I don't allow myself to think about what I am about to do, I find myself sitting in a dressing room in RTÉ studios with Kieran, doing everything I can to distract myself from the nerves. Usually I don't get nervous over interviews, but this is a whole other level that I am not used to. I pace up and down, telling myself it is only a conversation with someone, if I can just blur out everything else –

Freddie: *Are you talking about the live audience or the cameras or all the people watching you at home?*

'Not now, Freddie. You need to be on your absolute best behaviour tonight.'

Freddie: *I'll think about it.*

'You do that.'

I met Michelle at the hotel earlier when Kim came to wish us luck. The first thing I noticed about Michelle is that she literally doesn't give a fuck about anything. If she thinks something, she says it; she is honest, upfront and really doesn't like the word schizophrenia. She even went back years later and got a formal letter stating she is not to be classed as having schizophrenia any more. She embraces the voices she hears fully and accepts them as allies. She has names for most of them and openly talks about this. Meanwhile, I still keep Freddie to myself. He doesn't seem to care whether I speak about him out loud or not, he's just happy to be along for the ride. He loves Michelle and says something about her head sounding like a better place to be than mine.

A researcher goes through the questions with us in the green room. The subject of children comes up, and with it the stigma around people with schizophrenia becoming parents. The question which might or might not be asked is about whether Kieran and I are considering if there would be any problems with what I have. The truth is, it is on the cards. Kieran has wanted a child for years but I have always been unsure. I don't know if I would be a good mother – not because I have schizophrenia but because I can be a bit of a disaster and I just about manage to look after myself at the best of times. But since losing my own mother I have been thinking about it more. 'I know someone who got her children taken off her because she told the doctor she was hearing voices,' Michelle says. Lovely. I could have done without knowing that.

Freddie: *You leave my Michelle alone. Honesty is the best policy.*

Before I know it, it is time to go on. Kieran hides in the

green room because he doesn't want to get called on for a question if he sits in the audience. He is quite camera shy; he did the documentary without complaint for my sake but live television is a step too far for him.

We spoke to Ryan Tubridy, the host, backstage already before the show started. I was on his radio show years ago and I can honestly say he is the nicest person who has ever interviewed me. Probably because he is the same person and treats you the same both on and off air. That is not the case with a lot of them.

I hear a loud voice, the Geordie woman, as soon as Ryan asks me the first question, which throws me for a second, but I get back on track. Freddie stays quiet at least.

They do a simulation, similar to the one I did with the sound engineer in the documentary where different sounds I hear are played over the speakers, so the audience can get a taste of the type of noise in my head. Ryan asks how I cope with listening to that all the time and I ask him how he copes listening to the nothing sound I heard that one time when the voices stopped. Once it is over, I cannot believe I did it.

Freddie: *I actually thought you were shit but that's just my opinion.*

***

We finally go on our rescheduled honeymoon to America, which is the best time I have had in years. A few days after coming home I go back to the States again, to Texas, to meet my newborn niece, Jamie and Louise's daughter. They are living in Austin now because of Jamie's work. I am proud, to say the least. Lucy is gorgeous and perfect in every way. I had sort of forgotten, while more of our family passed away and our numbers dwindled, that it is possible to bring more additions into the world by creating them yourself. A baby tends to bring lost family closer together, and I notice how she even looks a bit like Mam from certain angles.

Since getting married I am asked when the babies are coming on a near-constant basis. I recently went for a smear and the GP asked about my name change. She asked if, now I was married, the discussion about having a baby had come up. When I told her that it had, the doctor told me that, to be on the safe side, she would refer me to the clinic for an appointment. I had not been there in years; I agreed to go because I was not sure if I had a choice.

A couple of weeks later, I attended my appointment. I went in thinking I would be in and out in fifteen minutes; instead, I spent the best part of two hours talking about every aspect of my mental health and whether I was having unprotected sex or not. The two men who were assessing me had a little meeting about me in the next room, and I heard every word. They really need to do something about sound-proofing that place. I sat in front of the two of them once they finished and the main guy told me I seemed to be doing well but if I did become pregnant, I would have to come back again, which sounds worrying.

In Texas, I watch the newest member of our family as she

lies on the floor, kicking and cooing. I wonder what babies think about. I wonder what baby me thought about. I can't imagine I heard voices then and, if I did, would they have sounded like babies or adults?

Freddie's voice never matured beyond a certain point. He sounded childlike when I was small, and while his tone eventually deepened, he doesn't have a manly voice. If I had to put an age on him, I would say he sounds about eighteen now. I have no idea why that is. Most of my earliest memories include Freddie. Since I found out that the face-less man and the bad woman were real, old memories of mine have become clearer. Random moments pop into my head sometimes. I remember now how I gave Freddie his name. He was around so much I thought he deserved a title. My dad was talking to someone about Live Aid and he mentioned Freddie Mercury. I was too small to know who he was but I must have liked how the name sounded and thus the predominant voice in my head became Freddie.

None of the other voices are around or have stuck around as long as him, so maybe that is why I never named anyone else. I have always been ashamed of giving my imaginary friend a name but not so much now. At least I never started naming crows or shampoo bottles.

My psychosis is weird now. It is there. Freddie pops in and out along with a few other old familiar ones. I still hear the noises. I get delusions sometimes. Nothing alarming, though. Nothing that stops me from going about my life.

HOW TO BE MENTAL TIP 25

A mental health problem is only really an issue when it stops you from carrying on with your day-to-day life. Your illness might still be there but, as a general rule, you're good as long as it's not messing up your life. If you can still do the tasks that are required of you to be a regular member of society and you can human reasonably well then you fit nicely into the 'in recovery' category. It's a nice place to be.

When it comes to having a baby, though, what I am mainly worried about is if I am able to be a mother. Not because of schizophrenia, though; after all, I have managed to jump through every obstacle so far with that hanging over my head. I worry more about how I still can't tie my shoelaces properly or use a tin opener, how the most basic tasks continue to be impossible for me. My hands won't cooperate, my whole body is still uncoordinated as ever. And how will I manage without my own mother to show me the way? I know how to do a lot of the practical stuff, like changing nappies, but what if something is wrong? Like a high temperature or a rash. How the hell do you wean a baby?

I have this conversation with Louise, who says she is pretty sure she had never even *held* a baby before having Lucy. She seems to know what she is doing, or at least they are figuring it out. They are definitely doing a great job for two people who decided emigrating wasn't stressful enough so they threw a baby into the mix.

People always say the mothering instinct kicks in but what if it doesn't happen for me? I accidentally dropped Gary once when he was a baby. He was fine once he had gotten over the initial shock – I laugh about it with him now – but at the time I was traumatised. My dad, who witnessed the whole thing, told me it wasn't my fault and stayed surprisingly calm for someone who had just seen their baby face plant off the floor.

Another worry is what people would think. I know I shouldn't care about that, but this is new territory, so I really do. People might judge me like they did when I said I wasn't on medication. I think of what Michelle said about the girl she knows. What if my child gets the piss taken out of them at school because of me? What if their friends are not allowed to come over to our house to play because their mother has schizophrenia?

I worry about all of these things for months.

Chapter 21

Mental illness affects most aspects of your life in one way or another. Including your physical health. When I was in school, I used to get shooting pains in my arms whenever I was going through a particularly bad bout of depression. Your bones sort of ache sometimes. Headaches and nausea are common too. Then there is the pressing weight on your stomach and chest, as though someone is sitting on you – most people with anxiety can relate to this sensation.

Usually when I get sick, I assume the first signs of symptoms appearing must be connected to my mental health. You kind of start blaming everything on your mental illness, probably because it messes up most things in your life, so it becomes the main culprit whenever you don't feel right. And over the last few days I haven't been feeling well at all. I have been on my work placement at *The Irish Times*, desperately trying to come across professional while I feel like I am swaying on a boat most of the time.

I can't figure out exactly what is wrong with me, something just feels off. At first, I go with the usual, 'It must be my mental health' conclusion but no, all good there. Then I think it is stress related, as I am surrounded by journalists, real ones, and I have no idea if I am doing an okay job or not. I have been experiencing vivid dreams as well, the absolutely mental ones I used to have when I was on anti-psychotics.

Then, one morning back at home, while Kieran is getting ready for work, I slip into the toilet without saying anything. I watch the little screen flash until the word appears. I rush out to tell Kieran the news: I'm pregnant.

The reason I haven't realised it is all pregnancy related up to this point is because we have been trying for months and I got so used to taking negative tests that I thought it wasn't going to happen for us.

But no, I am actually pregnant.

The only thing that terrifies me now is something happening to the baby. I keep thinking it is all too good to be true. I am due in December, which might take the sting out of Mam's anniversary and turn it into a happy time again.

After a while I start to relax a bit more. The scary, what-could-happen thoughts are there but I manage to push them away as much as possible. I have an entirely new feeling now. It takes me some time to realise what is is. It is unfamiliar, entirely different from anything I have ever felt before. For the first time in my life, I am happy.

I never had much will to live. Not that I was suicidal all of the time but I definitely wasn't that bothered about dying. I used to think of suicide like a safety net – oh if this or that happens and I cannot cope I can always kill myself and be done with it all. Not now, though. Pregnant me is extra careful crossing the street, more cautious, more aware of dangers. I used to think I would die young, likely because a part of me didn't want to stick around for too long. Now I want to live until I'm old and grey. I want to watch my child grow up and be there for it all. I need to be careful; I need to look after myself both mentally and physically, so I stay around for as long as I can. I have a future filled with birthday parties, Santa Claus, holidays, Mother's Day, the first day of school, the last, grandchildren. My mind races ahead to all we have to look forward to.

I develop symphysis pubis dysfunction (SPD), which I am simply going to explain as a wonky pelvis, and I hobble around on crutches with my big bump. No one tells you about all the weird symptoms: how your nose can block up for the entire duration of the event, giving you no choice other than to turn into a mouth breather, but at the same time how your sense of smell can be similar to that of a bloodhound. I have spots worse than I ever had as a teenager, my gums bleed and all I want to eat is oranges. I gain all sorts of knowledge, like the importance of pelvic floor exercises, what an inverted nipple is and just how far projectile vomit can travel. My nights are even more sleepless than usual between restless legs and turning over becoming something that takes several YouTube tutorials to learn how to do. Crying over everything becomes an everyday occurrence. My biggest tantrum happens while out shopping for a large pair of men's trainers, as they are the only thing my swollen feet will fit into; it looks like I am wearing a pair of miniature canoes when I try them on. A woman approaches me to ask if I am okay, thinking some sort of terrible tragedy has befallen me and I have to tell her a pair of shoes are the cause of my upset. Even throughout the morning sickness, the aches and pains, I know it will be worth it in the end.

Apart from the tears over my clown feet, my mental health is in good shape. I have to check in with the clinic but it is not as bad as I first thought. They are only there to keep an eye on me and make sure everything is going alright, the same way it would be if I had a physical illness.

Due to a mild case of placenta previa, which means that the placenta is lying low in the uterus, I have extra scans and check-ups at the maternity ward. I watch someone zip through my file before stopping and glancing up at me. 'A history of psychosis?' We do this every single appointment and each time I take the postnatal depression leaflet with a forced smile. They talk about the chances of me developing this or even postnatal psychosis. I read about a woman with this condition before. She went out of the room to get something for her baby and when she came back there were two babies, and she had to figure out which one was the hallucination. They keep talking about what would happen if the voices were to come back. I stay silent for these parts. Everyone always assumes my psychosis is something that goes away until I have an 'episode', as if there is no possible way I could function if it was there consistently. I used to think there was something even more wrong with me because I didn't fit the linear terms schizophrenia is given by psychology textbooks. I don't care about that any more.

There are good parts when it comes to being pregnant. Strangers smile at you as you waddle along; everyone is generally kinder than usual and people ooh and aww at the bump. Mothers you don't even know will give you advice on remedies for your ailments, like love-heart sweets for heartburn.

It's a strange time; your body goes through many changes. It's a bit like puberty but everyone knows what is going on and comments on it. The kicks are indescribable. I get my first one the day we trade in Mam's beloved car, which I ended up with, for a more family-friendly vehicle. I am upset about the change because crying is my first language now, but before we go to hand over the keys, I feel my first flutter, which is more like tiny bubbles popping.

I feel close to Mam in a way that I haven't since she died. Every day a robin comes to see me. He sits on the windowsill and stares in at me; he even comes in once, which is less of a beautiful moment and more of a running around screaming in terror about how to get him back out scenario, but the sign gives me some comfort regardless.

I love watching my bump grow, knowing that I was once a bump and Mam must have felt like I do now. We find out we are having a boy. I always dreamed of my first being a boy so I am delighted with the news. We form our own special little bond through his kicks and wiggling around.

HOW TO BE MENTAL TIP 26

One day you will find something that makes it all worth it and you will be grateful you stuck around. You won't wish to go back and change any of your journey because it led you to this point. You will no longer experience regret about the paths that didn't work out. You realise you are exactly where you were always supposed to be.

The first sign of something being wrong is when my waters break. Kieran has come home early from work; we are standing outside our bedroom, evaluating my symptoms as best we can with what little we know about contractions, when I feel it happen. I will spare you as much of the gory details as possible but let's just say that the water is not water; it is another colour to what I was expecting entirely. I am two days overdue at this point.

I am not in labour yet so I have to be induced. The waters have meconium in them, which basically means baby could not hold it in and has done a poo in the womb. Which sounds both adorable and disgusting but is actually quite dangerous.

We get settled in the room and meet our midwife. The contractions start but they are not too bad. As they progress and get stronger, I am surprisingly alright with them. After a couple of puffs of gas and air I decide it's not for me. Talk of the epidural starts then. I don't have a birth plan beyond getting the baby out safely. I thought I would start screaming for drugs early on but I have had so much pain throughout the pregnancy that my pain threshold is through the roof so I don't feel like I need anything. But once it's pointed out to me that I am better off having an epidural now rather than later when it might be too late, I agree to go ahead with it.

The anaesthesiologist comes in with her giant needle. I have always heard horror stories about it but I don't mind injections. I think it might be linked to my self-harm problems but that kind of pain doesn't bother me. They show me a consent form with the risks. *None of that will happen to me*, I think.

Once it is administered, the doctor comes in to examine me. He asks me am I really writing a book. I tell him I'm trying. He asks will he be in it. Maybe we'll discuss this when your hand isn't inside of me.

Freddie is interested in what's going on.

Freddie: *Does that hurt?*

Freddie: *Ugh, does that not hurt when they do that?*

Freddie: *I'm never getting pregnant.*

We watched every episode of *One Born Every Minute* and *The Rotunda*. Some people told me it was a bad idea but if I had not watched those shows I wouldn't know what is happening; remembering all of the births I have seen go this way gives me some bit of reassurance.

Kieran lingers by the bed while a midwife examines me. I wonder if it's just my imagination that she seems to be paying more attention to me than I expected at this stage, especially when I can hear the sounds of babies being born in the ward.

It's the last thing I think before it happens. I don't even see her do it but I know what the sound of the alarm means. Someone is in trouble. When I see all the staff running into the room towards me, I realise that the someone is me.

I only have a second to look at Kieran and I know that he knows too. The baby has responded badly to the epidural and his heart rate is dropping. I do what I always do in any kind of traumatic situation and dissociate out of there as quickly as possible. It's good for something.

Freddie: *Hey it's okay.*

Freddie normally isn't this nice when something is going on.

Freddie: *Let's stay calm. You've done really well. I'm proud of you. Gold star. And gold star for baby when he comes out too, yeah?*

As I am wheeled in for an emergency caesarean section Freddie keeps talking to me.

Freddie: *Hey, hey guess what? I got your mom here. We're right here with you.*

I know babies don't always cry when they first come out, so I prepare myself for that. My teeth rattle and my body shakes. Kieran and the anaesthesiologist are all I can see by my side as my view is limited to the ceiling. She keeps spraying me with water to test if I can feel anything or not. I can hear all the people in the room. The lights are bright and I squint at them. I feel the sensation of the knife making the incision but no pain, there is pulling as they peal back the layers and then I can feel hands tugging and rooting at my insides.

Freddie: *Mom is real proud of you, kid; she's here watching, don't you worry.*

I feel one last big tug.

'Here he is!' someone shouts.

He cries right away. He's alright.

'Danny,' I gasp and the tears come.

My baby is here and he's okay. The midwives are angels for how enthusiastic they get, even though they do this all day. I hear them say he is huge. They show him to me for a second. All I can see is his big eyes. I didn't know a newborn could have eyes like his. Kieran and I both have big, brown eyes too but his are the most beautiful sight I have ever seen. I don't even properly take in the rest of him. They take him to be weighed and checked. I hear Kieran tell me he's nine pounds and eight ounces.

Then there is nothing. I can hear them all talking but I can't make out what is being said. As the nothing continues, I start to think something might be wrong. It's Kieran who tells me. It's his breathing. Kieran keeps his tone light but I know him well enough to sense he's hiding something. The midwife, the one who was with me when his heart rate dropped, says, 'Let Mum give him a quick kiss before you go.' She puts him up to my face, he's wrapped tightly in a blanket and between the oxygen masks she sort of bumps him off my face for a second and then he is gone.

Later, I am wheeled up in my bed to the maternity ward. I'm on a lot of pain relief so I am not really with it. Kieran is with Danny. It's weird that he is an actual person now, not just a dream inside my belly.

Freddie: *Danny James Wall, huh? It's no Freddie but it has a nice ring to it.*

'Kieran didn't like Freddie.'

Freddie: *Like you would have used it anyway.*

'Hey, Freddie,' I think a while later.

Freddie: *What's up, kid?*

'I know you didn't really see my mam. I know you just said it to try and make me feel better.'

Freddie: *You got me. I didn't know what else to do. Shit was crazy, all the blood and the panic and stuff.*

'It's okay, I understand why you pretended. I'm sure she was there, in her own way. I'm not mad at you or anything.'

Freddie: *Good, because I wouldn't care if you were.*

'Freddie.'

Freddie: *What now?*

'Thank you. For being there for me and for like being there whenever I really need you.'

Freddie: *Not like I can go anywhere else. It's me that's stuck with you. But I am your favourite, right?*

'Always.'

Chapter 22

The next day, I sit and watch all the people walk past the bed. The three other women in the room have their babies. They cry, the mothers fuss over them, people come to visit. I apparently have a baby too. His name is Danny. He was born yesterday. He is a little sick but he's here. And he is my baby. I tell myself this repeatedly, trying to get it to sink in, while I wait until I am well enough to meet him.

When that time finally arrives, Kieran pushes me down in a wheelchair. We wash our hands and put on the gowns. I am wheeled towards a ward. I take in the sign above the door: Intensive Care Unit. All I can see is machines and the incubators with lots of wires and the tiny babies attached to them. Kieran wheels me over to one of the tiny, sick babies.

'How do you know that's him?' I ask, staring at the little thing with all his wires and attachments, unsure. I only saw him for literally seconds last night and I am pretty sure this is someone else's baby we are looking at through the plastic.

Kieran puts his hand through the holes in the incubator to touch him. 'Don't!' I snap at him. What if that really is another person's child and Kieran isn't supposed to touch him? Or what if we didn't wash our hands enough and our germs kill him? Or her. I don't know who owns this baby but I would really like to find where Danny is right now.

I look around the room. Thankfully I am too immobile to run around the room, looking for my baby, because after much persuasion Kieran gets me to realise that this baby is Danny. It doesn't feel like it, though. Everyone told me you get this rush of love when your baby is born, they put it on your chest and you have an instant connection. Lots of mothers I know have tried to describe the feeling to me. I look at my baby, I even get brave enough to put my hand in and rub his cheek. I like this baby, no, I love him, genuinely, but am I not supposed to feel more than this?

I stare at him as he blows bubbles out of his mouth. Whenever we go down to see Danny, he seems to be doing better. We get to take him out and hold him. The first time I hold him in my arms I ignore the trail of wires coming out of him and look into his eyes. I remember seeing them when he was born. I think that is the moment I truly realise it's really him. We are shown how to change his nappy, which is difficult when he is still hooked up to equipment. He has his first change without me, his first feed, his first bath. One day we arrive down and he is lying there in a cot with nothing attached to him, no machines, no drips; he gazes up to the ceiling looking chilled out.

***

I am sitting on my bed in the ward. All the other women in the room are looking after their babies and, as usual, I don't know what to do with myself. A midwife comes to show them how to bath their babies, and I try to listen in so I know what to do when the time comes. Kieran has gone to get me a coffee. The last few days have been tough. I had to leave Danny earlier today to go to a surprise mental health assessment. I was so happy after seeing him without any medical equipment that my mood must have showed because the mental health professional said I seemed to be doing okay.

I'm not sure if I am. I don't know how long this detachment I have with Danny will last. I figure it is there because we were separated at his birth and we never got to do skin to skin. Maybe I have been distancing him from me on purpose so it would be easier if things went the other way and he didn't recover so quickly. Kieran walks in with my coffee in one hand, while the other is pushing a cot. I shout Danny's name and jump off the bed. He is here, with me; I didn't make him up. He is real and he is mine.

The girl across from me literally leaps out from behind her curtain. 'Oh my God. I'm so happy for you and I'm sorry I haven't talked to you before. You know the way you can hear everything in here, I've been following the whole story and I felt awful when my girl wouldn't stop crying and you didn't have your baby and I didn't want to make you feel bad. Look at him, he looks really healthy. Do you want a picture of all of you together? Go on, I'll take it.'

She takes a picture of us, our first family photo. I cannot remember that girl's name but meeting her was the first time I found out that one of the best parts of being a mum is the other mums.

Look, I won't bore you with too much of the mushy stuff. I know new parents gushing over how perfect their baby is can get annoying. But I wrote most of this book in the months after Danny was born. I relived some of the most significant events in my life, wrote about psychotic breakdowns, psychiatric wards and deaths in the family while simultaneously playing peek a boo. So, I think I deserve a minute to talk about how incredible the little human we created is.

Danny is everything. The most amazing, funny, clever baby, who makes my world a wonderful place in which to live. It is not easy, at first; the bonding takes a bit of time to kick in. I don't feel guilty about admitting that any more. Danny arrived in unusual circumstances; it is natural that it took me a little time. I remember coming home from hospital, in pain, tired and clueless. We kept saying to each other how we couldn't believe we could take him home, how were they letting two idiots like us walk out with a newborn? How could we be trusted with such a responsibility?

Someone said to me that it must seem impossible to contemplate being away from him but that it is okay to ask for a break: sometimes you just need a reprieve from the endless cycle of feed, change, repeat. It is normal to not want to be around your baby 24/7. No one would judge me if I needed to get away for a bit, pop into town, do some Christmas shopping and clear my head. There is nothing wrong with needing to be away from him for a while, they said. 'What if I don't want to be around him at all?' I thought. I didn't say it out loud but I beat myself up about thinking it for a long time.

Eleven days after Danny was born it is Mam's anniversary. I wake up to a Christmas song on the radio, the same one that played when I said goodbye to her. After Kieran goes to work, I sit with Danny asleep on my chest, watching his breathing. His back rising and falling.

It happens then. The rush of love they talk about. There is no other love like it, the one you feel for your child; before this moment I loved him and wanted to protect him, but this is so much more. Unconditional, limitless, eternal love.

HOW TO BE MENTAL TIP 27

Just because it doesn't happen right away, it doesn't mean it won't. Everyone has a different experience. I always loved Danny more than I had ever loved anyone, but the maternal instinct took a little longer to kick in. Postnatal mental illness can trick you into believing you are a bad mother because you don't feel the way you think you should. Having a baby is tough, the hardest thing I have ever done. It is never your fault if one of the side effects of giving birth affects your mental health. We don't blame ourselves for our stitches or C-section scars or back pains, so we shouldn't blame ourselves if our minds are in bad shape after either.

No one tells you how much you cry after having a baby. Soppy ad on the telly. Cry. Dropped the baby's soother. Cry. Someone visits with a thoughtful present. Cry. Takeaway gave you the wrong toppings on your pizza. Cry. Make the mistake of watching *The Lion King* on Christmas Eve. Hysterics. The baby blues are very real and I panic about them at first, convinced I am showing signs of postnatal depression. Surprisingly enough, I never get it. All the emotions you feel after having your baby are like a release of hormones. I know I am lucky to escape any kind of post (or pre) natal illness. I think about times in the past when my mental health was at its worst and I cannot imagine how hard it must be to look after a baby while feeling like that.

I do, however, have some PTSD symptoms initially. Every time I hear the sound of an alarm, I get sucked into a play-by-play of the birth in flashbacks, which become so vivid and real I think they will never stop, until they eventually do. I appreciate how lucky we were to have a positive outcome. Once I get over the detachment wobbly, my mental health goes the other way. It seems to get better with each passing month. I love Kieran and I always have; he is a huge reason I survived all those tough times and stayed alive, but Danny has given me more of a reason than ever to keep fighting. I never want to leave him without his mother. I want to experience everything motherhood has to offer and watching him grow has made my life worth living. Not that it isn't worth living in general. I am glad he helped me to realise how good life can be. This is the cheesiest thing I will ever say but what really saved me in the end was learning how to fall in love with being alive.

It is decided that I don't need any more treatment for now. And I must stress the *for now* of that sentence. Any checkups I had were in my best interest, and it is good to know help and support will be there for me if I need them in the future.

Being a mother is a tough job. It is relentlessly challenging and you don't get to clock off at the end of the day. Those first few months, between colic and reflux, there are days when we think we are failing. Just when you think you have the hang of things, baby has a bad day and you feel like the worst parent in the world. And there's the worry, the constant anxiousness. Checking 142 times a night that he is breathing, has he been fed enough, is he too warm, which quickly spirals into fretting over the fact that one day he is going to move out and leave me and oh god someone is probably going to break his heart at some point and there is nothing I will be able to do about it.

There is a lot more to parenthood than cute Instagram pictures. It is a wild ride, filled with emotion, funny moments, times when you want to run away and a constant competition over which one of you is more tired. I think I win because, despite what some people have said to me, having a baby does not cure insomnia. You are guaranteed sleepless nights with a newborn, the only difference is that when baby wakes at 3 a.m. for his bottle, I am already awake and waiting for him. This has led me to complete and utter exhaustion.

The first time we bring Danny to a restaurant there are a mother, a daughter and the daughter's newborn baby at the table beside us. The mother is asking the daughter how the baby slept last night. They talk about all the things new mothers talk about with their mams. I wonder if that woman knows how lucky she is to still have her mother. Danny has one less person in the world who adores him in that extra special way, who cares about the mundane parts of our day and his little milestones that might seem dull to other people. Mam wouldn't mind if I sent her endless photos of him every day with all the updates. I will always need her, even though she will never be here again, but I am doing okay, more than okay.

Becoming a mother has made me happier than I have ever been. I just wish she could be here to see it. I am proud of all the things I learned myself: how to feed him, change him, bathe him, what to do when he is sick. I taught myself all of the practical stuff. But the love, the cuddles, the laughs, that's all her; she showed me how to love and she showed me how to be strong. Her love only exists in my heart now, but I use it to be the best mother I can be.

Chapter 23

Depression still rolls around in my mind sometimes. Delusions try to get to me and I have to do a quick sanity check, pushing them out of my head so they cannot get to me any more. The voices I can live with. Anxiety gets to me the most but I have some control over it. I don't believe we should always focus on the positive. Life is not very positive; the negatives have to be acknowledged too.

For me it is more about choosing which thought to focus on. When I try to think more positively, good things tend to happen to me. Like with my list, I fairly ticked off those goals which may have seemed unachievable at the time. I have heard it said that people like me should not expect much from life, but I don't agree. You should aim as high as you want to; wonderful things happen when you have some belief in yourself. It is better to have an oops than a what if. None of it happened by chance, my little dreams happened because I *made* them happen.

I said before that the most important rule of surviving a mental health problem is to accept you have one but I think I need to change that now. Determination will get you through, more than anything. That's not to say it is easy. There will be a lot of days when you have zero motivation, when getting out of bed will seem like the greatest mountain to climb, and there is nothing wrong with that. Being mentally ill will zap your energy, drain your emotions and leave you feeling like a sack of shit; after all, you are fighting a battle that has left you broken, but the energy needed to fix yourself will come, as will the motivation. Of course, having some determination doesn't mean you will live each day bouncing around, making lists, exercising, eating well, meditating and going to therapy to feel better. Sometimes determination can be lying in bed, needing a shower, procrastinating from your responsibilities while hiding away from the world. If, somewhere deep in your mind, you think, 'This is one bad day, not a bad life, someday soon I will be in a better place', that is determination, that is being motivated. The fight is still in you, even if being in the bad place is overshadowing it right now.

There was this salon I used to work at, where one of the regulars was being seen by someone else while I sat at the reception desk. She was telling my co-worker about her sister who had been recently diagnosed with bipolar disorder. I will never forget the words she used, as I furiously live messaged them to Kieran because I was so pissed off. 'See I just don't understand that way of living. My thinking is, go out and have a run; these mental problems are excuses because you don't like how your life is going. How do you expect your life to be if you stay like this?' My heart went out to her sister. I know only too well what it is like to have some family members who don't get it but who *think* they do.

The thing about being mentally ill is that everyone has an opinion on what should make you better. Live, laugh, love, go out and get some fresh air, improve your diet, take up a hobby, do some mindfulness, get to the gym. Mentally ill people are not stupid, we all know what is helpful. Getting well enough to do it, however, is another story. If it was that easy to overcome, none of us would ever be sick.

People with mental health problems don't go around walking into walls and scratching their heads, waiting for someone with a 'Positive Vibes Only' T-shirt to give them advice on getting better. We all know the steps needed to maintain good mental health but when you have spent three weeks inside your house, curled up in a ball sobbing your heart out, words of wisdom from someone whose entire knowledge of mental health comes from watching a storyline on *Coronation Street* are not much help.

Stay with me here because I am about to sound exactly like one of those people, but at least I know the struggle. Happiness is a choice. I know, I hate using such a bullshit phrase but I swear there is truth in it. You do whatever you have to do to get out of the bad place; every small change to your lifestyle counts. If you couldn't get out of bed at all yesterday but today you got up, changed the sheets, had a shower and then went back to bed, then that is progress. If you change your way of thinking even the teeny tiniest bit, leaning towards the good rather than the bad, that one baby step is better than nothing. You don't wake up one day, decide to be happy and suddenly everything is wonderful – but making that decision, that you are going to try your best to be happy, is the first step. Even if your best might feel shit in comparison to someone else's. No matter how small your best is it is always good enough. You are good enough. But remember that depression is an illness, not a mentality; therefore, the 'happiness is a choice' rule won't apply until you are past the worst point of it.

I know getting help can be incredibly difficult. Our mental health service is severely lacking: more needs to be done. While this is true, we need to do our bit too. We need to care about our own and everyone else's mental health more, not just on days dedicated to suicide prevention. We can post all the inspirational quotes and helpline numbers we want during mental health awareness month, but it is meaningless if we don't stop treating each other badly both online and in real life.

'It's okay not to be okay' is 100% true but there is no point in saying it only when it suits you and your personal situation, then throw that mantra out the window when it comes to someone famous or somebody you don't know personally. Posting some 'Copy and paste this if you are always here to listen' is useless if you are going to laugh at someone with bipolar disorder having a manic episode. Don't do Darkness into Light if you secretly make fake profiles to troll people online. Wearing a green ribbon is irrelevant if you are going to tell your friend with depression to get over themselves. It is perfectly fine to dislike someone, we all have people we cannot abide, but you don't need to shout about it online. You don't need to share the meme making fun of the overweight person, you don't need to screenshot someone's Instagram post to laugh at with your mates in a group chat, you don't need to drag a person down for expressing their passion for something you think is silly.

Life is shite sometimes. A television programme, a comic book, dressing up in a costume, jigsaw puzzles, crosswords, make-up, Morris dancing – whatever it is that makes a person happy and brings a little joy into their life should be celebrated. You should never take the piss out of someone for having interests, it could be the only good thing that gets them though a crappy day.

If you wouldn't say it to someone in real life, don't say it online. If you don't like someone, it is not necessary to inform them. Don't forget about the real person with feelings on the other side of your remark. You never know what someone is going through. You cannot judge someone's entire life based on their social media; we usually only post the good moments anyway because we put far too much effort trying to *appear* happy to strangers online instead of actually enjoying life. You can choose to be kind and your day will continue as normal. Resisting the urge to be mean won't kill you, but your being nasty might just kill them.

You might think I am being dramatic, but if you ask anyone who has contemplated or attempted suicide, you will learn that one cruel remark can send you over the edge, while one kind gesture can literally save your life by giving you a tiny bit of hope that it isn't all bad.

And that is the truth. Not everything is bad, even if it might seem like it sometimes. There is so much good in the world. Most people have good in them. You have to look closely to see it in some but it is there. If being open about mental health has taught me one thing, it is that people care about each other's well-being. We want everyone to be in the good place, we don't want people to suffer. We may not know how to help and we are all guilty of not knowing what the right thing to say is. People can come across as miserable and hateful but it is usually because they are going through something and their anger is misplaced. Of course, horrible people exist, but the majority of us are making the best possible choices we can based on our life experience so far. I find that helps me to forgive. Take my friends who turned against me after I came out of hospital, for example. It might seem like what they did to me was awful but I can see now how they were just making the best decision they could based on what knowledge and experience they had at the time.

I look back at all the things I could have done differently. Things might have gone better if I had gone straight into pursuing media after school, but then that would not have stopped me from getting sick. I could have waited to go to Australia but then maybe I wouldn't have achieved the goals I set for myself or I would not have had Danny. Life has a funny way of working itself out. I can forgive myself now for mistakes made in the past, people I should have treated better (including myself), situations I could have avoided, because without them I wouldn't be the person I am today. And as much as I annoy myself at times, I don't hate myself any more. I am a different person than I used to be.

If you don't like who you are or where you are at, remember you are who you are until you're not. Something will happen along the way that is going to either change who you are, making you a better person, or help you to realise that there was nothing wrong with who you were all along.

Epilogue

Freddie is good – though we had a falling out recently after he recited a poem that he wrote about me that was far from complimentary. This is my first time telling Freddie's story. He is difficult to sum up in an interview or a short article; I needed the space of a book to do him justice. He also doesn't actually like me talking about him; he gets angry about it for some reason. I have long since given up trying to understand him and who he is. Freddie might come across like a cool sidekick sometimes but, in reality, there is a lot of random chatter to wade through before I can understand what he is actually saying. I am grateful for him, though; I don't know how my life would have turned out without him. That's something I don't even try to imagine any more.

My psychosis has become something I find as manageable as a tickly cough or a hangnail irritating but it does not regularly impact my overall health. I have decided to go and get an assessment as an adult and see what the deal is with the learning difficulties, motor skill challenges, face blindness, etc. I would like to finally understand and make sense of those problems. Particularly when it comes to the face blindness, as not recognising people's faces comes with a lot of challenges. It is no easy task to explain to someone that I didn't neglect to salute them out of rudeness, that instead I just have no idea what they look like.

Some of the issues I spoke about having earlier may seem like they never got a conclusion, but that is because they remain unresolved. I am still very much a work in progress. I had to leave some holes in my story, certain experiences that I am not ready to share yet. I still have bad days, a lot of bad days, but we are good for the most part.

Speaking of doing well, Gary has really turned his life around. He still has a way to go but he has come along so much. He has made something of himself and left the bad stuff behind him. I could not be prouder of him. He has been a fantastic uncle and a great support to me. It has been a tough journey for him, as his life went on hold after the brain injury: he had to watch all the people around him get on with things while he was stuck. The accident took away so much from him and it is only now the real Gary has come back to us.

Jamie and Louise ended up moving back to Ireland. They have had another baby, Anna. Those two little girls have brought so much happiness to everyone. We all live close by; we might not be the closest of families but we have our individual relationships with each other, which I think is the best we can hope for right now. It's easy to have a happy family when things are going right; when the shit hits the fan and your world falls apart, you all have to make the effort for it to work.

Shelia passed away after the two younger babies were born. I am glad that at least she got to meet Danny. My dad met someone the year after my mam died. He has remarried and is moving away. He seems happy with his new life.

I can never come up with a straightforward answer to how I manage to be high functioning. I guess that is because it is a combination of different things. I think my schizophrenia must be mild compared to others. The fact that I no longer have bad voices has a lot to do with it. How long I have lived with this is a huge factor; as I have said before, psychosis is my normal.

If you are in the bad place, I would hate it if my story has negatively impacted your recovery in any way. And I want to remind you that you should never compare your journey with someone else's. What worked for me may not do the same for you. I think it is important that I tell you how some parts of this book made me sick, while reliving some moments sparked off some symptoms that I had not experienced in a long time. Having said that, I'm glad I went there, as writing about some of my worst moments helped me heal from wounds I didn't know were so big in the first place. I have also realised the ways in which I need to change, identifying aspects of my personality on which I need to work to become a better version of myself.

I don't think there is anyone out there, no matter how neurotypical their brain is, who can say they have never been to the bad place. Everyone has something going on in their lives, whether it be big or small. My problems and your problems might seem like nothing in comparison to someone else's ,but all problems are relevant; there will always be someone who has it worse. As much as I may have overused the word throughout this story, none of us is really normal; we all have a little crazy inside of us and there is nothing wrong with that. Everyone has their moments in the bad place; the only differences between us are the reasons we got there and the ways in which we get out. No matter what, we all need a bit of extra help sometimes, we all need to talk. Whether you have good mental health and need to maintain it, or you need help with ill mental health, this aspect is just as important as our physical health.

My wish for you is that you find whatever it is that makes it all worth it. I hope you find peace inside your mind. We all have our battles; everyone has that one thing that hurts them more than anything. Whether it is something temporary, or you lost something that you can never replace, I hope you find a way to be happy through the pain. It's okay to be sad, there is no shame in feeling the way you feel. Pain is part of being human.

No matter what happened in my life, I used to have this invisible kind of magic inside me that kept me going, something that made me feel hopeful even when I may not have had much reason to be. I used to say it was the hope that made it so much harder, because it would never allow me to truly give up, even though I desperately wanted to sometimes. That hope probably saved me in the end. Don't give up before it gets better. Even if your whole world falls apart, what you are going through now will one day become a story of how you overcame the worst part of your life and, you never know, it could help someone going through the same thing.

And no matter what, you are never alone. Those of us with mental health problems are everywhere. It is important for both ourselves and others that we do not hide our mental health away and let it be a heavily stigmatised, taboo subject. There are so many of us going through the same thing. We meet people every day who are fighting the same fight as us. The world can be a cruel place and we are all just trying to navigate it while keeping some of our sanity intact.

And there you have it. I hope you got something from reading my story. I would especially love if it made you feel something and, most of all, I hope it helped you in some way. I am sorry if it made you sad at any point. I don't see my journey as any kind of sob story, though. I feel I am lucky with the life I have had so far; I think it has been quite a good one. There were bumps in the road but I made it through. As the saying goes, life is tough but so are you.

I also apologise for the cheesy bits. I like to take inspiration from other people's words, I know how silly that might sound but remember what I said about letting people enjoy the things that make their day better? This applies here. My favourite quote of all time is from J. K. Rowling: 'Happiness can be found in the darkest of times if one only remembers to turn on the light'. I think that fits how I feel about it all. There is happiness to be found. Kieran didn't give it to me; any success I have had didn't give me it either; even the little human jumping beside me in his bouncer so enthusiastically as I write this that I fear he will take flight at any moment did not provide happiness for me. It came from within, when I made the decision to put more energy into appreciating these wonderful people and things I have in my life. I realise now that my life is pretty amazing. I can find joy in the little things and somewhere along the way I learned how to be me.

If I could say anything to my younger self it would be to hang in there, it doesn't stay bad forever; one morning you are going to get up, make breakfast and sit watching cartoons with the two loves of your life and it will all be okay. It might look like a boring life to some people. Kieran works in a supermarket, I stay at home with Danny, and we are broke most of the time. I cook, I clean, I change nappies, I write whenever I can, we hardly ever have the energy to go out, Saturday nights consist of falling asleep in front of the TV. But it is a lot more perfect than I ever could have imagined and to complete our little family baby number two is on the way and we are very excited about her.

My story is far from over. I know there will be many times in the future where I will end up in the bad place again but, for now, I am going to appreciate being well and not worry about what might be around the corner. I feel the next time I get sick might not be as bad, because I know what it is like now to be on the other side of things: the good place. And let me tell you, it was all so worth it.

I never thought I would get here; life really is mad.

Acknowledgements

And here it is, the part I was dreading because I'm not very good at telling people how I feel about them, but I will give it my best shot. First and foremost, to you, the reader: it means more to me than you will ever know that you chose to read my story. It is a story that could not have possibly come together without the help of my mother-in-law/chief babysitter, Breda. Thank you for everything you do. To Sue and Johnny: I would be lost without you; thank you for kind of adopting me. A huge thank you to Sylvia, my one-woman support system and mammy number 2. George's Court crew – my weird and wonderful best friends – I love each and every one of you; thank you for existing. Gary, there are no words to express how proud I am of you, and to your Katie – thank you for coming into our lives and making it a brighter place. And of course a shout-out to the rest of the family: Jamie, Louise, Lucy, Anna, Sherree, Dean, David, Fionnuala, Liam, Suzanne, Noel and Aoife. Tony, thank you for all the support. I will always love you.

Thank you to the incredible team at Mercier Press for making this possible and giving me the opportunity to share my story. Patrick, I am so glad you found me; I can never thank you enough for this. To all the teachers who showed me patience and kindness – Colette O'Mahony, Pat Knightly, Michael O'Sullivan, Martyna Coffey, Antoinette O'Brien, Tina Hunt and Michelle Daly. Thank you to all the mental health warriors I have met along the way. You are a huge part of my story. You welcomed me into this community, inspired me and showed me what being strong really is. Included in this is the late Seán O'Reilly, an amazing person who always encouraged me to keep writing. I wish more people got to read his story. I would also like to mention the kind internet strangers who follow Pretty Sane on social media – thank you for all the love, support and words of encouragement. It means the absolute world to me.

And finally, to the most important people. Ishy (sorry for calling you Kieran), I can't believe I am lucky enough to spend my life with you. Thank you for keeping me mild-to-moderately sane as I wrote this, while we also learned how to be parents at the same time. Thank you for cheering me on, making me laugh, for always believing in me, for never doubting me and my crazy dreams, and for loving me long before I learned how to love myself. Danny, one day you will be old enough to read this and when that time comes I am sure you will already know this, but I want to tell you that I have never loved anyone or anything as much as I love you. You saved me, baby boy. The world is a wonderful place with you and your dad and bump in it. You are my everything.